INFECTIOUS DIARRHEAL DISEASES

MICROBIOLOGY SERIES

Series Editors

ALLEN I. LASKIN
EXXON Research and Engineering Company
Linden, New Jersey

RICHARD I. MATELES
Stauffer Chemical Company
Westport, Connecticut

Volume 1 Bacterial Membranes and Walls
edited by Loretta Leive

Volume 2 Eucaryotic Microbes as Model Developmental Systems
edited by Danton H. O'Day and Paul A. Horgen

Volume 3 Microorganisms and Minerals
edited by Eugene D. Weinberg

Volume 4 Bacterial Transport
edited by Barry P. Rosen

Volume 5 Microbial Testers: Probing Carcinogenesis
edited by I. Cecil Felkner

Volume 6 Virus Infections: Modern Concepts and Status
edited by Lloyd C. Olson

Volume 7 Methods in Environmental Virology
edited by Charles P. Gerba and Sagar M. Goyal

Volume 8 Microtubules in Microorganisms
edited by Piero Cappuccinelli and N. Ronald Morris

Volume 9 Handbook of Indigenous Fermented Foods
edited by Keith H. Steinkraus

Volume 10 Unusual Microorganisms: Gram-Negative Fastidious Species *edited by Edward J. Bottone*

Volume 11 Laboratory Manual for Medical Microbiology *edited by The Faculty of the Department of Microbiology, Schools of Medicine and Dentistry, State University of New York at Buffalo*

Volume 12 Infectious Diarrheal Diseases: Current Concepts and Laboratory Procedures *edited by Paul D. Ellner*

Other Volumes in Preparation

INFECTIOUS DIARRHEAL DISEASES

Current Concepts and Laboratory Procedures

Edited by

Paul D. Ellner

The Presbyterian Hospital
and
College of Physicians and Surgeons
Columbia University
New York, New York

MARCEL DEKKER, INC. New York and Basel

Library of Congress Cataloging in Publication Data

Main entry under title:

Infectious diarrheal diseases.

(Microbiology series ; v. 12)
Includes index.
Contents: Campylobacter enteritis / Martin J. Blaser -- Yersinia enterocolitica / Edward J. Bottone -- Non-cholera Vibrio gastroenteritis / Don J. Brenner -- [etc.]
1. Diarrhea. I. Ellner, Paul D. (Paul Daniel) II. Series. [DNLM: 1. Diarrhea--Etiology--Congresses. 2. Diarrhea--Microbiology--Congresses. 3. Communicable diseases--Etiology--Congresses. 4. Communicable diseases--Microbiology--Congresses. 5. Diagnosis, laboratory--Methods--Congresses. W1 MI292S v.12 / WI 407 I43]
QR201.D4I54 1984 616.3'427 83-23131
ISBN 0-8247-7129-X

MARCEL DEKKER, INC.
270 Madison Avenue, New York, New York 10016

Current printing (last digit):
10 9 8 7 6 5 4 3 2 1

PRINTED IN THE UNITED STATES OF AMERICA

Preface

Diarrheal diseases constitute the largest single cause of death in the developing nations where a child has a fifty percent chance of dying before the age of seven.....primarily from a diarrheal disease. Such diseases are not limited to the developing countries; in the United States, diarrhea ranks high among the principal causes of death of young children.

Until relatively recently, infectious diarrhea was considered to be due almost exclusively to *Salmonella, Shigella, Vibrio cholerae,* or intestinal parasites. Within the past decade or so there has come the recognition that other genera can cause diarrhea as well: *Campylobacter fetus* ss *jejuni, Yersinia enterocolitica,* non-cholera halophilic vibrios such as *Vibrio parahaemolyticus, Clostridium perfringens, Bacillus cereus, Clostridium difficile,* enteropathogenic strains of *E. coli,* and certain viruses. Epidemiologic studies have revealed that some of these organisms, particularly *E. coli* and *Campylobacter,* may account for a larger percentage of diarrheal disease in some populations than *Salmonella* and *Shigella* combined.

There are at least two rather different syndromes having diarrhea in common; the "small bowel syndrome" characterized by profuse watery diarrhea leading to dehydration and electrolyte imbalance, and the "dysentery-colitis syndrome" associated with fever, intestinal inflammation, and possible pseudomembrane formation. Research on the pathogenesis of diarrheal diseases has demonstrated that there are several mechanisms that may be involved, including the production of enterotoxins, cytotoxins, alteration of the villi, or invasion.

The therapy of diarrheal diseases depends upon the specific etiologic agent and consequently the clinical laboratory may be called upon to detect and identify these pathogens. Understanding the pathogenesis of diarrheal diseases is the first step leading to rational therapy. It is well established that fluid and electrolyte replacement may be life-saving in small bowel syndromes like cholera. The potential hazards of disturbing the intestinal commensal flora or using drugs that reduce intestinal motility is now recognized. In the future, treatment or even prevention of some diarrheas may be accomplished by the ingestion of innocuous substances that interfere with the attachment of some of these pathogens.

This volume had its genesis from a symposium which dealt with developments in the laboratory diagnosis of bacterial diarrheas. It soon became obvious that a book dealing solely with laboratory procedures would have a limited value, and consequently, the material was expanded to include aspects of epidemiology, pathogenetic mechanisms, and non-bacterial agents as well.

The overall philosophy of the book has been to select etiologic agents about which detailed information has been derived fairly recently, and have this information discussed in depth. It is hoped that this book will provide a source of such information useful to microbiologists, physicians, and perhaps, students of medicine.

I wish to acknowledge the assistance of Mrs. Mary Lou Ramm, whose help in maintaining contact between the contributors, editor, and publisher was extremely helpful.

Paul D. Ellner, Ph.D.

Contents

Contributors

NEIL R. BLACKLOW, M.D., Division of Infectious Diseases, University of Massachusetts Medical School, Worcester, Massachusetts

MARTIN J. BLASER, M.D.,* Division of Bacterial Diseases, Center for Infectious Diseases, Centers for Disease Control, Atlanta, Georgia

EDWARD J. BOTTONE, Ph.D., Department of Microbiology, The Mount Sinai Hospital, New York, New York

DON J. BRENNER, Ph.D., Division of Bacterial Diseases, Center for Infectious Diseases, Centers for Disease Control, Atlanta, Georgia

GEORGE CUKOR, Ph.D., Division of Infectious Diseases, University of Massachusetts Medical School, Worcester, Massachusetts

ROBERT FEKETY, M.D., Division of Infectious Diseases, Department of Internal Medicine, University of Michigan Medical School University Hospital, Ann Arbor, Michigan

JOHN D. FRAME, M.D., Division of Tropical Medicine, School of Public Health, Columbia University College of Physicians and Surgeons, New York, New York

*Current affiliation: Division of Infectious Diseases, Department of Medicine, University of Colorado School of Medicine, Denver, Colorado.

ALEX C. SONNENWIRTH, Ph.D., Departments of Microbiology and Immunology, and Pathology, Washington University School of Medicine, Division of Microbiology, The Jewish Hospital of St. Louis, St. Louis, Missouri

ALEXANDER von GRAEVENITZ, M.D., Department of Medical Microbiology, University of Zurich, Zurich, Switzerland

KAYE WACHSMUTH, Ph.D., Molecular Biology Laboratory, Bacterial Disease Division, Center for Infectious Diseases, Centers for Disease Control, Atlanta, Georgia

INFECTIOUS DIARRHEAL DISEASES

1

Campylobacter Enteritis

MARTIN J. BLASER*
Division of Bacterial Diseases
Center for Infectious Diseases
Centers for Disease Control
Atlanta, Georgia

Presented as part of the symposium "Recent developments in the laboratory diagnosis of diarrheal diseases" at the 80th Annual Meeting of the American Society for Microbiology, Miami Beach, May 13, 1980.

Campylobacter jejuni was, until recently, quite obscure to most clinical microbiologists. What follows, then, is an overview of the recent work on *Campylobacter*. For more specific information the reader is advised to consult the accompanying references (1-4).

Figure 1 gives a schematic representation of the genus *Campylobacter*. *Campylobacter* belongs in the family *Spirillaceae* (3). The

*Current affiliation: Division of Infectious Diseases, Department of Medicine, University of Colorado School of Medicine, Denver, Colorado.

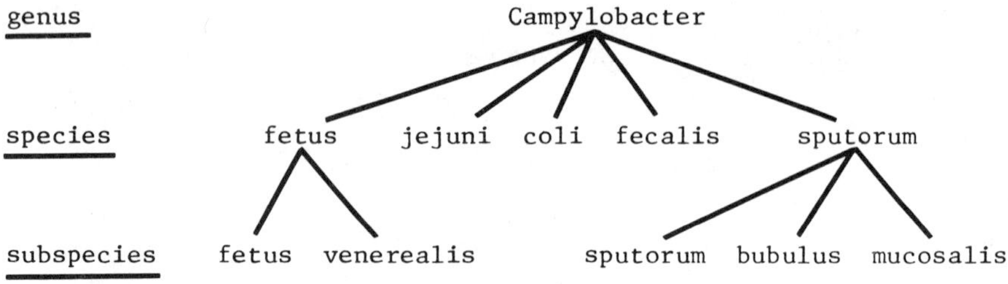

Fig. 1 The genus *Campylobacter*.

genus *Campylobacter* consists of 4 species: *C. fetus, C. jejuni, C. sputorum,* and *C. fecalis*. Closely related to *C. jejuni* is *C. coli* which is now considered to be a separate species. Because of their biochemical and epidemiologic similarities, these organisms can be considered as one and referred to collectively as *C. jejuni*.

C. fetus and *C. sputorum* each have several subspecies. At the present time, only *C. fetus* subsp. *fetus* and *C. jejuni* have been recognized as human pathogens; because of the infrequency of infection due to *C. fetus* subsp. *fetus*, this discussion will focus on *C. jejuni*. The nomenclature of the campylobacters has changed several times and the older literature may include different terms; the present terms appear to be based on a solid scientific foundation (5).

Figure 2 shows a gram stain of a pure culture of *C. jejuni*. Carbol fuchsin was used as the counterstain because campylobacter are poorly stained by safranin. The organisms are gram-negative, slender, spiral, or curved rods. They can also appear as S-shapes and as gullwings. In cultures more than 48 hours old coccoid forms predominate.

To understand the importance of *Campylobacter* to clinical microbiology, one must understand the history of this organism. *Vibrio*-like organisms were first isolated from aborted calves in 1909 and called *Vibrio fetus*. Similar organisms were found to infect sheep, swine, and fowl; however, it was not until 1947 that the

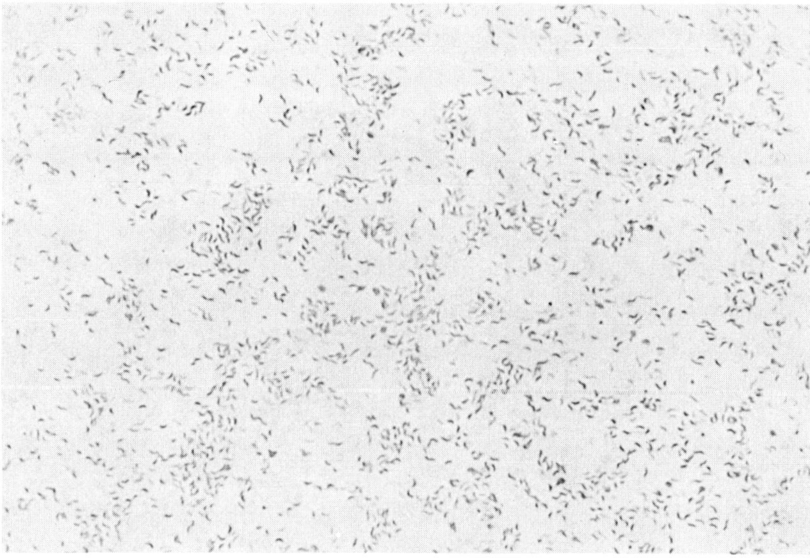

Fig. 2 Gram stain of 48-hour culture of *C. jejuni*.

first human infection with *Vibrio fetus* was recognized. Most early isolates were from debilitated hosts, but in 1957 Elizabeth King observed that certain isolates from patients were atypical, and each isolate was assocated with diarrheal disease (6). These organisms she called "related vibrios," and we now know them as *Campylobacter jejuni* and *Campylobacter coli*. However, they were fastitidous and could not be isolated from stools until selective methods were employed. In the past 10 years, investigators around the world have used such methods and have now isolated *Campylobacter* from the stools of patients with diarrhea.

During these past 10 years, the prevalence of isolation of *Campylobacter* in persons with diarrhea and in healthy controls has been studied (Tables 1 and 2) (7-10). *Campylobacter* was isolated from 3% to 12% of the stools of patients with diarrhea in these investigations. These percentages approximate or exceed the isolation

Table 1. Isolation of *Campylobacter jejuni* from Patients with Diarrhea and from Healthy Controls

Investigator	Place-year	No. of Subjects	% with Campylobacter	No. of Controls	% with Campylobacter
Butzler	Belgium-1973	900	5.0	1,000	1.3
Skirrow	England-1977	803	7.1	194	0
DeMol	Rwanda-1978	204	10.8	58	0
Pai	Canada-1978	1,004	4.3	176	0
Blaser	U.S.A.-1978	514	5.0	157	0
Steele	Australia-1978	224	5.8	540	0

Table 2. Relative Frequency of Isolation of *Campylobacter* Species From Humans

C. jejuni	*C. fetus* subsp *fetus*
Isolated on all 6 continents (12,000 cases in U.K. in 1982 alone)	200 cases in the world's literature
Pathogen of healthy hosts	"Opportunistic" pathogen
Recovery from stools: 3-12% in patients with diarrhea	Rarely recovered
Belgian study (22,000 patients): 5.9% recovery in patients with with diarrhea	3 cases (.01%)

rates for *Salmonella* or *Shigella* in these same populations. Among asymptomatic individuals, however, isolation was very uncommon. However, in the developing countries the epidemiology of *Campylobacter* infection appears to be different (11). Healthy children have been found to be infected as frequently as children with diarrhea. Whether this finding represents asymptomatic infection in the healthy children or long term carriage following a diarrheal episode is not known. The relationship of infection to specific immunity may provide an answer to these questions.

Based on these considerations, the next important question to answer is whether *Campylobacter* is indeed a pathogen for man? Some of the evidence that it is may be summarized as follows: In developed countries, it is commonly isolated from patients with diarrhea, but only rarely from asymptomatic individuals. It is a known pathogen for sheep and cattle. Some patients have had isolations simultaneously from diarrheal stools and from the blood stream. When tissue has been available for histologic examination, the acute exudative inflammatory reaction has resembled the pathologic conditions described in animals (6). Infected patients have been shown to have rising antibody titers to their isolate. Recently 2 volunteers ingested campylobacter organisms in glasses of milk, contracted a typical illness, and *Campylobacter* was isolated from their stools (10,12). The increasing number of outbreaks of enteric illness in previously normal individuals from whom *Campylobacter* is isolated provides further support for its pathogenicity. In total then, a substantial body of evidence has been accumulated showing that *C. jejuni* is a human enteric pathogen (1).

Although human infection with *C. fetus* subsp. *fetus* is well recognized, it will be reviewed only briefly (Table 2). Whereas there have been tens of thousands of isolates of *C. jejuni*, the cases of *C. fetus* infection have been few. *C. jejuni* apparently can affect anyone; *C. fetus* appears to be largely an opportunistic organism affecting debilitated hosts. Whereas *C. jejuni* is frequently recovered from the stools of diarrheal patients, *C. fetus* rarely is. For example, in a large survey in Belgium, *C. jejuni* was isolated from 5.9% of patients with diarrhea but *C. fetus* was isolated from only 0.01% (13).

The epidemiology of *Campylobacter* infection seems to resemble that of *Salmonella* (14). Animals appear to be the major reservoir for *Campylobacter* in nature. Transmission of infection to humans has occurred after direct animal-to-human contact, after ingestion of contaminated milk and water, and by person-to-person spread. However, ingestion of contaminated food and water are believed to be the leading modes of transmission. All ages have been affected by *Campylobacter* infection, and there is a summer peak in the incidence of isolation.

The target organs of infection are both the large and small intestine; however, the relative frequency of involvement of each is not known. Infection produces an acute exudative and hemorrhagic inflammation. Stools frequently contain both blood and leucocytes. The pathophysiology of the infection is not known, but most evidence suggests tissue invasion as the mechanism (1,2).

Most assessments of campylobacter infection have included patients who presented to a hospital with diarrhea (7-10). Our understanding of the clinical infection is thus mostly limited to patients with diarrheal disease. The course of the diarrheal illness observed has been quite variable. Infected individuals may have mild symptoms or no symptoms at all. Frequently, infection is expressed as an illness of 2-7 days' duration characterized by diarrhea, abdominal cramps, and constitutional symptoms such as fever, malaise, and muscle aches. Campylobacter enteritis may mimic either a viral gastroenteritis or acute salmonellosis or shigellosis. At the more severe end of the spectrum, illness with bloody diarrhea, fever, and severe abdominal pain has been noted. These manifestations may mimic acute appendicitis or acute ulcerative colitis. Fatalities, although rare, have been reported.

In general, however, the clinical course of campylobacter enteritis lasts 1 week or less in most patients. When antimicrobial treatment is clinically indicated, erythromycin and tetracycline appear to be the agents of choice. However, most patients improve spontaneously. Relapse may occur but long-term sequelae appear to be uncommon.

Presentation of the salient epidemiologic and clinical features of campylobacter infection leads to the next question: How can *Campylobacter* be isolated and identified in the clinical laboratory? Isolation is the major obstacle; however, there are 4 key principles for success in isolating *Campylobacter:*

1. The specimen should be plated shortly after being obtained, or kept refrigerated in an appropriate transport medium;
2. The plating medium should be sufficiently rich to support the growth of *Campylobacter*;
3. The medium should be selective to inhibit growth of the normal stool flora; and
4. The atmosphere should be microaerobic to permit growth of *Campylobacter*.

Each of these 4 main points will now be reviewed.

Campylobacter does not survive well in stool specimens or rectal swabs left at room temperature for more than 24 hours. Specimens should be refrigerated or transported to the laboratory in an appropriate transport medium. When kept refrigerated, Cary-Blair, Stuart's and Campy-thio, a modified thioglycollate medium containing antibiotics, all permit survival of organisms for more than 1 week (15). Because organisms do not survive well in buffered glycerol saline, its use is not recommended. Phase contrast microscopy of *fresh* stools from ill individuals may show typical darting forms, and gram stains may show vibrio forms; these are specific diagnostic aids but the sensitivity of each is about 50-70% (16,17).

For isolation of *Campylobacter* from stools, a rich medium is optimal. Brucella agar, Columbia agar, Oxoid Blood agar base #2, and Thioglycollate agar have proved useful in the past. Enrichment with 5% blood also improves recovery, but more than 5% is not necessary. In pure cultures *Campylobacter* will grow on blood agar plates with a typticase soy base, but this is not recommended for isolation from stools.

Such rich media, however, will also support the growth of the normal enteric flora. Historically, elimination of this flora was first done with filtration; however, this is a cumbersome procedure for most clinical laboratories. An easier method is to incorporate into the media antimicrobial agents that will selectively inhibit the background flora. Three such media have been widely used: Skirrow's (2), Butzler's (2), and Campy-BAP (9). Each of these has a potent array of antimicrobial agents to inhibit stool organisms. The question as to which of these media is most satisfactory in clinical laboratories is currently undergoing study. Certain *Campylobacter*-like organisms may be susceptible to the antibiotics in these media. Another means of selection is by incubating plates at 42°C. *C. jejuni*, but not other campylobacters, grows optimally at this temperature, and many enteric organisms will be inhibited at 42°C.

Campylobacters are by definition microaerophilic although there is variability within the genus in the degree of oxygen tolerance. They will not grow in the ambient atmosphere, and optimal growth occurs at about 5% to 6% oxygen. Providing an appropriate level of oxygen for incubation is critical. Augmenting the carbon dioxide concentration in the atmosphere has been recommended but is not critical. Both of these conditions can be met by using vacuum jars, partially evacuating them, and then refilling them with a mixture of nitrogen and carbon dioxide. Another method that has been employed is to use Gas-Paks (BBL Microbiology Systems, Cockeysville, MD)* without the catalyst. Because this results in liberation of free hydrogen, which has explosive potential, this method should *not* be used. Commercial companies (BBL, Oxoid Ltd.) have now developed campylobacter-specific gas generating packets which have eliminated this problem. Candle jars that lower the oxygen level to 17% are not as sensitive for recovering small concentrations of *Campylobacter* from stool as vacuum jars that maintain 6% oxygen. However, considering the high concentration of organisms in most diarrheal stools (18), this may not be a problem: studies by Wang and colleagues suggest that incubation of clinical specimens in candle jars may be nearly as sensitive as in 6% oxygen, provided that incubation is at 42°C. Another method suggested for providing an appropriate atmosphere is in the use of the Fortner principle (19). This method employs facultative aerobes to consume the oxygen in a closed environment, thus lowering the oxygen concentration. However, this method is cumbersome for most laboratories and is not recommended. Another method reported is the use of prereduced media, such as George's ferric sulfate, sodium metabisulfite, pyruvate (FBP) medium (20). The utility of this method must be tested in clinical situations.

When these 4 steps are followed, correct transport, use of a rich base, use of selective conditions, and a reduced oxygen concentration for incubation, the isolation of *Campylobacter* is not difficult. Plates should be incubated for 48 hours; when a candle

---

*Use of trade names is for identification only and does not indicate endorsement by the Department of Health and Human Services or the Public Health Service.

jar is used, incubation should be for up to 72 hours. Figure 3 shows the colonial morphology of a pure culture of *Campylobacter*. Note the 4+ growth of these characteristic grey, mucoid, nonhemolytic colonies.

A rapid presumptive identification can be made with the following characteristics: 1. typical colonial morphology, 2. typical Gram stain showing gram negative curved rods, 3. indication of oxidase and catalase positivity, and 4. motility. Organisms that grow under the selective conditions and meet these criteria will be finally identified as *C. jejuni* or a closely related species at least 98% of the time. In the interest of brevity, the remaining tests for confirming the identification will not be presented here but these are widely available (3).

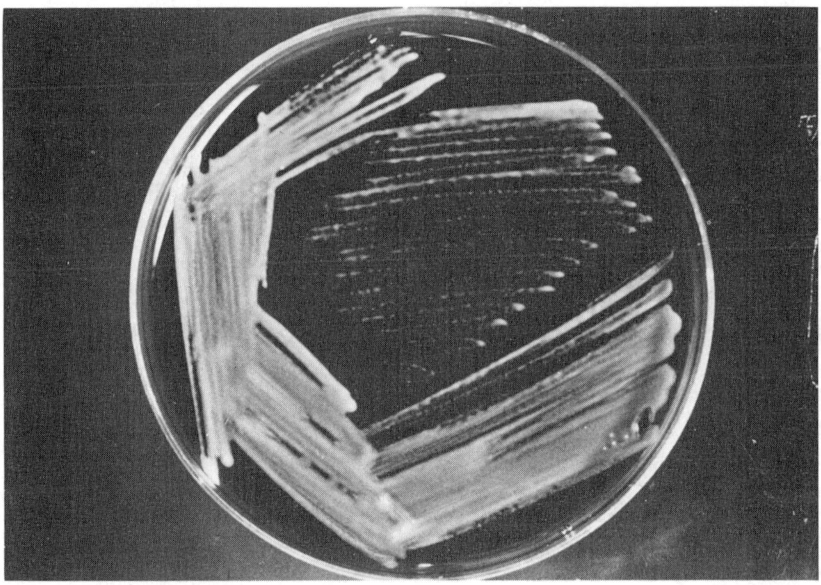

Fig. 3 Pure culture of *Campylobacter jejuni* incubated at 42°C for 48 hours on brain-heart infusion agar with rabbit blood.

In summary, *Campylobacter jejuni* is an important cause of diarrheal disease throughout the world and is as or more commonly isolated as either *Salmonella* or *Shigella*. Usually infection appears to cause gastrointestinal and constitutional symptoms that last for less than a week. *C. jejuni* can be easily isolated from clinical specimens when selective media are incubated in an appropriate atmosphere.

ACKNOWLEDGMENT

The author thanks Dr. Wen-Lan L. Wang, in whose laboratory the stimulation to work on this fascinating microorganism first began.

REFERENCES

1. Blaser, M. J. and Reller, L. B., *Campylobacter* enteritis. *N. Engl. J. Med., 305:*1444-52 (1981).
2. Butzler, J. P. and Skirrow, M. B., Campylobacter enteritis. *Clin. Gastroenterol, 8:*737-65 (1979).
3. Smibert, R. M., Part 6. Spiral and curved bacteria. In: Buchanan, R. E. and Gibbons, N. E., eds. *Bergey's Manual of Determinative Bacteriology*. 8th ed. Baltimore: Williams and Wilkins Co., 1974, pp. 207-12.
4. Smibert, R. M., The genus *Campylobacter*. *Ann. Rev. Microbiol., 32:*674-709 (1978).
5. Skerman V. B. D., McGowan, V., and Sneath P. H. A., Approved lists of bacterial names. *Int. J. Syst. Bacteriol., 30:*225-420 (1980).
6. King, E. O., The laboratory recognition of *Vibrio fetus* and a closely related vibrio isolated from cases of human vibriosis. *Annual N.Y. Acad. Sci., 98:*700-11 (1962).
7. Demol, P. and Bosmans, E., Campylobacter enteritis in Central Africa. *Lancet 1:*604 (1978).
8. Pai, C. H., Sorger, S., Lackman, L., Sinai, R. E., and Markks, M. I., Campylobacter gastroenteritis in children. *J. Pediatr., 94:*589-91 (1979).

9. Blaser, M. J., Berkowitz, I. D., LaForce, F. M., Cravens, J., Reller, L. B., and Wang, W-L. L., Campylobacter enteritis: clinical and epidemiologic features. *Ann. Intern. Med., 91:*179-85 (1979).

10. Steele, T. W. and McDermott, S., Campylobacter enteritis in South Australia. *Med. J. Aust., 2:*404-06 (1978).

11. Bokkenheuser, V. D., Richardson, N. J., Bryner, J. H., et al., Detection of enteric campylobacteriosis in children. *J. Clin. Microbiol., 9:*227-32 (1979).

12. Robinson, D. A., Infective dose of *Campylobacter jejuni* in milk. *Br. Med. J., 282:*1584 (1981).

13. Lauwers, S., DeBoek, M., and Butzler, J. P., *Campylobacter* enteritis in Brussels. *Lancet, 1:*604-05 (1978).

14. Blaser, M. J., LaForce, F. M., Wilson, N. A., and Wang, W-L. L., Reservoirs for human campylobacteriosis. *J. Infect. Dis., 141:*665-9 (1980).

15. Luechtefeld, N. W., Wang, W-L. L., Blaser, M. J., and Reller, L. B., Evaluation of transport and storage techniques for isolation of *Campylobacter fetus* subsp. *jejuni* from turkey cecal specimens. *J. Clin. Microbiol., 13:*438-43 (1981).

16. Paisley, J. W., Mirrett, S., Lauer, B. A., Roe, M., and Reller, L. B., Darkfield microscopy of human feces for the presumptive diagnosis of *Campylobacter* enteritis. *J. Clin. Microbiol., 15:*61-3 (1982).

17. Sazie, E. S. M. and Titus, A. E., Rapid diagnosis of *Campylobacter* enteritis. *Ann. Intern. Med., 96:*62-3 (1982).

18. Blaser, M. J., Hardesty, H. L., Powers, B., and Wang, W-L. L., Survival of *Campylobacter fetus* subsp. *jejuni* in biological milieus. *J. Clin. Microbiol., 11:*309-13 (1980).

19. Karmali, M. A. and Fleming, P. C., Application of the Fortner principle to isolation of *Campylobacter* from stools. *J. Clin. Microbiol., 10:*245-8 (1979).

20. George, H. A., Hoffman, P. S., Smibert, R. M., and Krieg, N. R., Improved media for growth and aerotolerance of *Campylobacter fetus*. *J. Clin. Microbiol., 8:*36-41 (1978).

2

Yersinia Enterocolitica

EDWARD J. BOTTONE
Department of Microbiology
The Mount Sinai Hospital
New York, New York

When considering the evolution of members of the genus *Yersinia*, one immediately conjures up visions of the plague bacillus (*Yersinia pestis*) decimating in its wake vast populations of 18th century Europeans. In the recess of bacteriological evolution one also encounters the magnificent description by Malassez and Vignal in 1888 (35) of yet another yersinial species the "pseudotuberculosis" bacterium, (*Yersinia pseudotuberculosis*). Today, however, our interest has been focalized on the third; a "newcomer", chronologically documented in the 20th century (1939) by Schleifstein and Coleman (47), the bacterium of enterocolitis, *Yersinia enterocolitica*.

Interest in *Y. enterocolitica* among a substantial interdisciplinary cross-section of medical food and veterinary scientists, epidemiologists, taxonomists, and physicians derives from a singular event which occurred in 1976 in the upper New York State hamlet of Holland Patient. In this tranquil setting, *Y. enterocolitica* emerged as the focal point of intensive activity as the causative agent of an epidemic gastroenteritis involving 222 subjects. Reports of the outbreak were first brought to the public through two newspaper accounts (Figures 1,2) each presenting the data in their own inimical style. These articles documented that 12 (later 16) children had undergone appendectomies for what was subsequently recognized as "yersinosis enterocolitica".

Prior to the formal published report of this outbreak (6) only 61 cases of *Y. enterocolitica* infection had been reported in the United States since its first description in 1939 (47). Interestingly, none were reported for nearly 30 years until 1968 when Sonnenwirth (50) described a patient with *Y. enterocolitica* bacteremia and meningitis and subsequently re-emphasized the importance of this microorganism as a human pathogen (51). In Europe, however by 1976 over 5000 isolates has been collected at the Pasteur Institute most originating from the Scandinavian countries (H. H. Mollaret, Personal Communication).

Historically, the nomenclature of any given microorganism usually unfolds through a variety of imaginative terms bearing the designator's reference point. Thus, the microorganism named *Y. enterocolitica* in 1964 by Frederiksen (24), had previously borne epithets like *Pasteurella X* (19), *Pasteurella pseudotuberculosis* type b (20), *Bacterium enterocoliticum* (48), and Les germes X (37). Indeed, while it was recognized that *Y. enterocolitica* was related to *Y. pseudotuberculosis*, there was little agreement as to what comprised *Y. enterocolitica*. The mainstay of such confusion arose

THE NEW YORK TIMES, THURSDAY, OCTOBER 21, 1976

12 Undergo Appendicitis Operation For Ailment Calling for Antibiotics

HOLLAND PATENT, N.Y., Oct. 20 (AP) —A dozen youngsters here who have had emergency appendectomies in the last three weeks did not hav appendicitis at all, but a rare intestinal disease with the same symptoms, physicians reported today.

State Health Department officials said the children had been stricken by a disease known as yersiniosis, after the genus Yersinig, and which is caused by a highly contagious bacteria.

They said they believed a contaminated water system in this central New York village was responsible for what they called the most severe recorded outbreak of the disease.

Residents here were told in August to boil their drinking water because of a water treatment system described by state health officials as "primitive."

One doctor defended the surgery, saying it would have been "too dangerous" to have ignored the symptoms.

"In the judgment of the people who saw the patients initially, they all had the symptoms of appendicitis," said Dr. Daniel Stowens, director of the laboratory at St. Luke's Hospital in Utica, about 15 miles south of Holland Patent. Dr. Stowens said his hospital had handled five or six cases of illness from the Holland Patent area. "It was only after two or three of them turned out not to have been appendicitis that the suspicion [of yersiniosis] dawned."

Surgeons also performed three or four emergency appendectomies on children at City Hospital in nearby Rome, according to a hospital pathologist who declined to be identified. He said the hospital's laboratory later isolated yersiniosis bacteria in the patients' stools.

At least 30 people, mostly children, have come down with the illness in Holland Patent, according to Dr. Kenneth MacLeod, the Oneida County Health Commissioner. He said the symptoms included fever, vomiting, diarrhea and skin rashes —symptoms similar to those of appendicitis.

Holland Patent, a village of 600 people, was named for Henry Lord Holland, who received a grant, or patent, of 20,000 acres of land from the British Government in 1769.

Epidemiologists from the State Health Department are interviewing people who had symptoms of the disease, asking them what they have eaten and drunk, and where they have been during the last month.

Dr. Stowens said the patients' symptoms were "clinically indistinguishable" from appendicitis.

A dammed-up, stream-fed pool, which provides the water for Holland Patent, flows through a pasture in which cows and horses graze, resulting in the possibility of bacteria from animal wastes entering the system, health officials said.

Fig. 1 New York Times account of Holland Patent outbreak of *Yersinia enterocolitica* gastroenteritis.

Was Knife Needed?

12 Children Were Misdiagnosed

Holland Patent, N.Y. (Special)—As many as 12 children who had a fever and were vomiting underwent emergency surgery for removal of their appendixes in the last three weeks in hospitals in Utica and Rome. Physicians said yesterday that the children did not have appendicitis, that they had an intestinal disease with similar symptoms.

Officials of the State Health Department said they believe that a contaminated water system was responsible for the disease.

Officials said a dammed-up, stream-fed pool provides the water for this village in central New York. The stream flows through a pasture in which cows and horses graze, raising the possibility that bacteria from animal wastes had got into the water. All of the children live here and drank water from the system.

Residents of this village of 600 had been told in August to boil their drinking water because of a water treatment system described by New York State officials as "primitive." The only treatment for the local water supply is chlorination.

"You're just about drinking raw water," said Dr. Richard Jackson, a State Health Department epidemiologist.

The school system replaced tap water with bottled water at the beginning of the school term for 2,000 children in three schools. But the suspected water remained available from several sources, including bathroom sinks.

Experts of the State Health Department said the disease was yersiniosis, an ailment caused by a highly contagious type of bacteria.

A lively medical debate broke out yesterday about the appendicitis operations that were performed on children in St. Luke's Hospital in Utica, 15 miles south of Holland Patent, and at City Hospital in nearby Rome.

Dr. Daniel Stowens, director of the lab at St. Luke's Hospital, said it would have been "too dangerous" to ignore the symptoms of the disease — fever, vomiting, diarrhea and skin rashes.

A pathologist at City Hospital in Rome who asked that his name not be used said yersiniosis bacteria had been found in the stools of patients after surgeons there performed three or four emergency appendectomies on children.

A spokesman for the State Health Department said the agency was not investigating the question of whether the appendectomies should have been performed.

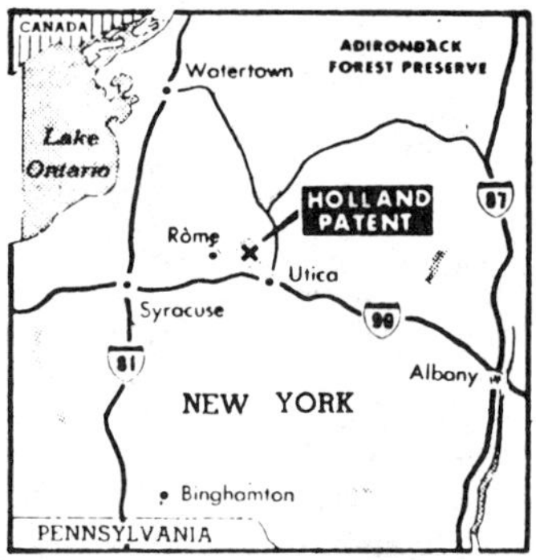

News Map by Bill Kresse

Central upstate area where children were hit by intestinal disorder.

Fig. 2 New York Daily News account of Holland Patent outbreak of *Yersinia enterocolitica* gastroenteritis. (Reprinted by special permission from New York News Inc. 1976.)

because of the biochemical heterogeneity of strains designated *Y. enterocolitica*. Isolates with unifying characteristics for inclusion as *Y. enterocolitica* (Table 1) also displayed variability regarding several other features including indole production and rhamnose fermentation.

Retrospectively, Van Loghen in 1944 (57) proposed the genus name *Yersinia*, to include *Y. pestis* and *Y. pseudotuberculosis*, formerly classified in the genus *Pasteurella*. Thal in 1954 (52), placed the genus *Yersinia* in the family *Enterobacteriaceae*, and Frederiksen in 1964 (21) after examining 55 strains bearing many of the aforementioned appelations, showed that these species were distinct from *Y. pseudotuberculosis* but allied enough to warrant placement in the genus *Yersinia* as a separate species *Y. enterocolitica*.

In 1972 Knapp and Thal (30) posed the question "What is *Yersinia enterocolitica*"? showing the species was a conglomerate of strains deviating in many biochemical aspects. They recognized the four groups as shown in Table 2, which also appends their conclusions. Subsequently, a great degree of order was brought to *Yersinia* taxonomy largely through the efforts of Brenner (14,15) who, using biochemical characteristics and DNA/DNA hybridization studies, recognized the four species of *Yersinia* designated in Table 3.

Typical Y. enterocolitica (Group 1). These strains are uniform in their biochemical and serological parameters and, along with *Y. pseudotuberculosis*, comprise the major pathogens for man and animal. Among such strains are the "classic" serotypes comprising O-antigen groups O:3, O:5,27, O:8, and O:9, which account for the majority of human infections. These serogroups contain both indole positive and negative (O:3) strains.

Rhamnose fermenting strains (Groups 2,3).

Rhamnose positive, raffinose, melibiose and α-methylglucoside negative isolates have been shown by Brenner to be distinct from typical *Y. enterocolitica* from which they differ only in rhamnose

Table 1. Distinguishing Characteristics of *Yersinia* Species*

Test	Yersinia			
	Pseudotuberculosis	Enterocolitica	Intermedia	Kristensenii
TSI Slant/butt	alkaline/acid	acid/acid	acid/acid	alkaline/acid
KIA Slant/butt	alkaline/acid	alkaline/acid	alkaline/acid	alkaline/acid
Motility 22°C	+	+	+	+
37°C	0	0	0	0
Urease	+	+	+	+
Oxidase	0	0	0	0
Lysine decarboxylase	0	0	0	0
Arginine dihydrolase	0	0	0	0
Phenylalanine deaminase	0	0	0	0
Simmons citrate	0	0	+(22°C) or 0	0
Indole	0	V	+	+(22°C)
B-galactosidase	+(22°C)	+(22°C)	+(22°C)	+ or 0
Acetylmethylcarbinol 22°C	0(V + L)	+	+	0
37°C	0	0	0	0
Ornithine decarboxylase	0	+	+	+ or 0
Fermentation:				
Glucose	+	+	+	+
Lactose	0	0	0(+L)	0
Sucrose	0	+	+	0
Rhamnose	+	0	+(22°C)	0
Raffinose	0	0	+(22°C)	0
Melibiose	+	0	+(22°C)	0
α-Methyl glucoside	0	0	+(22°C)	0
Trehalose	+	+, 0	+	+ or 0

Y. frederiksenii differ from typical *Y. enterocolitica* only by rhamnose fermentation. 0 = negative, + = positive, (+L) = late positive, V = variable.

Table 2. Division of *Yersinia enterocolitica* into 4 Groups (Knapp and Thal, 1972)

Group	Indole	Xylose	Esculin	Salicin
1. *Y. enterocolitica* Pasteurella "X"	0	V	0	0
2. *Y. enterocolitica* Pasteurella "X"	V	+	0	0
3. Esculin + Salicin +	+	+	+	+
4. Lactose + Rhamnose + Sucrose 0	V	V	V	V

"We propose for indole negative strains the species name *Y. enteritidis* and for the indole positive strains, *Y. enterocolitica*".

"Strains of groups 3 and 4 do not belong to the species *Y. enterocolitica*."

Table 3. Speciation of *Yersinia* Based on Deoxyribonucleic Acid Hybridization Studies and Biochemical Reactions*

Species	Representative Serotype(s)	DNA Homology Group	Biochemical Characteristics
Y. enterocolitica	0:3;0:5,27	I	Typical, Indole positive and Indole negative strains
*Y. frederiksenii**	0:16	II	Rhamnose positive, raffinose, melibiose α-methyl glucoside negative
*Y. intermedia**	0:17;NAG$^+$	III	Rhamnose, raffinose melibiose, α-methyl glucoside positive
*Y. kristensenii***	0:11;0:12	IV	Typical-except for negative sucrose fermentation and Voges-Proskauer test.

*Brenner (15,16).

**Species name being proposed (D. J. Brenner, Personal communication)

NAG$^+$ = nonagglutinable.

fermentation. The name *Y. frederiksenii* has been proposed for these isolates in honor of Dr. W. Frederiksen (56a).

Rhamnose, raffinose, melibiose and α-methyl-glucoside fermenting isolates (Group 3) comprise a heterogeneous collection of strains enjoined by DNA homology and the above distinctive biochemical attributes. These strains are mainly of environmental origin. The name *Y. intermedia* has been proposed for such isolates (14a) as they share biochemical and antigenic properties with both *Y. enterocolitica* and *Y. pseudotuberculosis* (3,7,9,17).

Group 4. Sucrose and acetylmethylcarbinol (Voges-Proskauer) negative and trehalose fermenting isolates comprise DNA-homology Group 4 of Brenner. Such isolates differ from typical *Y. enterocolitica* by the two listed features. The name *Y. kristensenii* has been proposed for these species (4a).

The ascription of distinct species status to the variety of organisms formerly classified as *Y. enterocolitica* has clear clinical and epidemiologic significance. Through subsequent studies regarding virulence factors (see below), it is now known that members of Groups 2, 3, and 4 are mainly derived from the environment, lack invasive potential, and have not been associated with the classic syndromes e.g., mesenteric lymphadenitis, terminal ileitis, acute gastroenteritis, and septicemia (8,10,38). The new species designation clearly delineates the pathogenic potential inherent in the designation *Y. enterocolitica* and affords a reference point for distinguishing the nonpathogenicity of the new species.

I. LABORATORY IDENTIFICATION

Morphologically, when observed in direct smears of an exudate, *Y. enterocolitica* presents as a gram-negative, *Pasteurella*-like coccobacillus with somewhat rounded ends (Figure 3). When viewed after growth on artificial media, the observed morphology is more

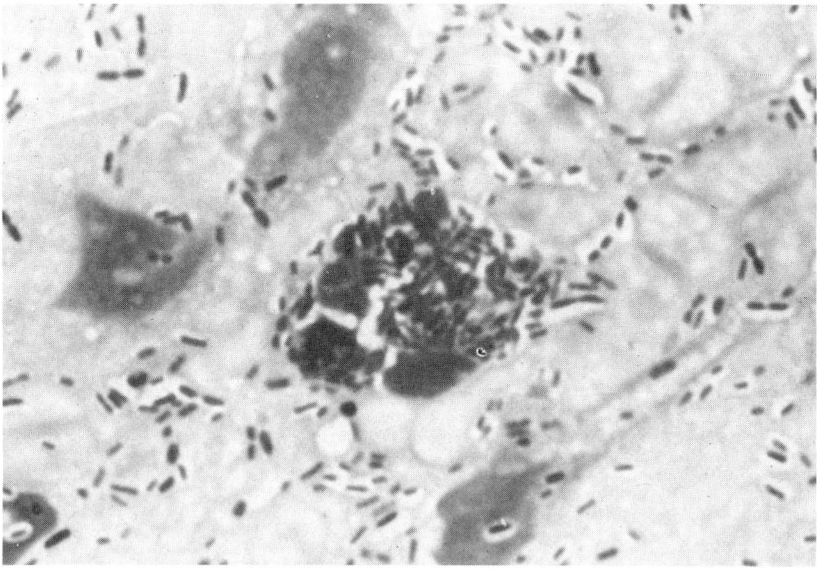

Fig. 3 Gram-stain smear of *Yersinia enterocolitica* from peritoneal exudate of experimentally infected laboratory animal (mouse) showing bacillary to cocco-bacillary (some encapsulated) morphology.

consistent with that of *Enterobacteriaceae* as bacillary forms and filaments predominate.

The laboratory diagnosis of *Y. enterocolitica* requires an exquisite appreciation for the temperature-related biologic phenomena associated with this species. As shown in Figure 4, affected by growth at lower incubation temperatures (22-25°C) are numerous surface-related interactions which include synthesis of antigens necessary for adherence to, and penetration of, epithelial cells (31,55) resistance to intracellular killing and serum bactericidal activity, altered phage susceptibility, lowering of LD_{50} doses (40), and serologic reactivity. Regarding the latter, in the author's laboratory we have observed that the sera of patients with *Y. enterocolitica* bacteremia reacted faintly in agglutination tests with their own isolate used as an antigen after growth at 37°C.

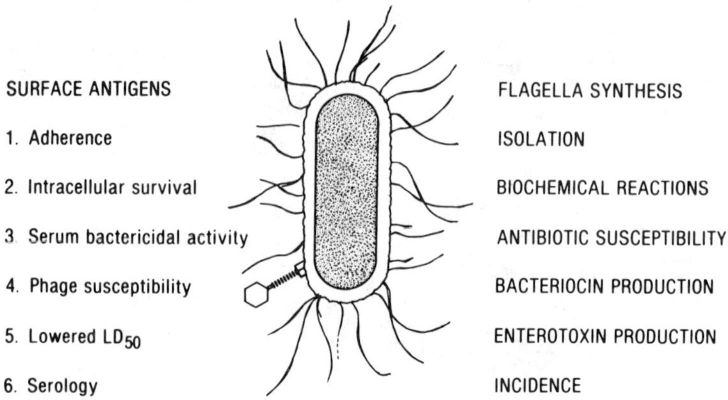

Fig. 4 Biologic attributes of *Yersinia enterocolitica* expressed after or affected by growth at 22°C-25°C (see text).

In contrast, the same sera produced strong agglutination (1:1024) of the homologous isolate after growth at 22°C (11a).

Other important temperature-related attributes germane to isolation, identification and pathogenesis, include cold (4°C) enrichment, various biochemical reactions (Table 1), flagella synthesis (25°C), bacteriocin production among *Y. intermedia* isolates (11), enterotoxin production (41) and tissue invasiveness (65).

Culturally the recovery of *Y. enterocolitica* from grossly contaminated samples such as feces requires an awareness of the pinpoint aspect of colonies and their "color" reactions on a variety of commonly used "enteric" agar media. These are depicted in Table 4. In order to maximize recovery of *Y. enterocolitica* and related species from stool specimens, several media may be inoculated in duplicate followed by incubation at 25°C and 37°C respectively. Alternatively one set of media may be inoculated, incubated at 37° overnight, and then at 25°C for an additional 24-48 hours. While *Salmonella-Shigella* (SS) agar favors growth of serotypes 0:3 and 0:9, the inclusion of MacConkey agar will enable recovery of other serotypes as well as other *Yersinia* species which may be inhibited

Table 4. Colonial Tinctorial Characteristics of Classic *Y. enterocolitica* on Commonly Used Enteric Media

Agar Medium	Colony Size[b]		Colony Color
	25°C	37°C	
Deoxycholate (DC)	Pinpoint	0.05-1 mm	Colorless
Endo	0.05-1 mm	0.05-1.5 mm	Colorless
Eosin methylene blue (EMB)	Pinpoint	Pinpoint	Lavender (24 hr) metallic sheen (48 hr)
Hektoen-enteric (H-E)[a]	Pinpoint	Pinpoint	Salmon
MacConkey	Pinpoint	1.5 2 mm	Pinkish hue
Salmonella-Shigella[a] (SS)	Pinpoint-0.05 mm	Pinpoint-0.05 mm	Colorless
Xylose-lysine[a] deoxycholate (XLD)	Pinpoint	Pinpoint	Yellow; irregular edges

[a]*Y. intermedia* strains grow poorly or not at all on these media.
[b]24 hours incubation at 25 and 37°C.

on SS agar. Recently (Table 5), selective and differential agar media have been developed to enhance the recovery of *Y. enterocolitica* from stool specimens. Using stock cultures von Riesen (60) reported on the ability of *Y. enterocolitica, Y. pseudotuberculosis* and *Y. pestis* to digest polypectate (polygalacturonic acid) incorporated into an agar medium producing as a result depressed colonies. Bowen and Kominos (12) subsequently extended these observations to include three rhamnose fermenting strains as well. The characteristic sinking of *Y. enterocolitica* colonies into the agar depths (Figure 4A) served to distinguish this species from among numerous other *Enterobacteriaceae* thus enhancing isolation. Clinical evaluation of this medium will enable further assessment of pectin agar for the recognition of *Yersinia* species.

A second cultural innovation designed to enable the early presumptive identification of *Y. enterocolitica* was introduced by

Table 5. Selective and Differential Media for Recovery of *Yersinia Enterocolitica*

Author	Medium	Discriminating Reaction	Comment
Lee, 1977	Tween-80-MacConkey	Tween-80 hydrolysis zone of precipitate,	Variable reaction among classic strains.
Juhlin, 1961	LSU Agar	Lactose-sucrose fermentation, urea hydrolysis.	Colonies develop slowly.
Dudley-Shotts, 1979	CAL	Cellobiose-arginine-lysine	Burgundy colonies, cellobiose fermentation. 0.5-1.0 mm pinpoint red center. 4 isolates colorless.
Bowen-Kominos, 1979	Pectin agar	Pectin digestion depressed-colonies (0.7% agar).	Colonies easy to distinguish. *Klebsiella oxytoca* also gives depressed colonies.
Schiemann, 1979	CIN agar	Cefsulodin, irgasan, novobiocin	*Yersinia* colonies red (mannitol fermentation), highly selective.

Dudley and Shotts (21). These investigators added cellobiose, arginine and lysine (CAL), along with other ingredients to an agar matrix. As *Y. enterocolitica* ferments cellobiose, an acid pH is rendered which imparts to the colonies a burgundy or red coloration. While this medium was effective in distinguishing 20 of 22 isolates, two *Y. enterocolitica* strains failed to elicit the desired reaction as they were cellobiose-negative. The medium, which according to these investigators was as sensitive as MacConkey agar for recovery of *Y. enterocolitica*, was not tested for recovery of and differentiation of rhamnose-positive or sucrose-negative isolates.

Schiemann (46) has reported on the value of a medium he devised (CIN agar) for the discrimination of *Y. enterocolitica* from most other gram-negative species capable of growth on this medium. The selective aspect was conferred by incorporating cefsulodin, irgasan (2,4,4'-trichloro-2'-hydroxy diphenyl ether), and novobiocin, while the differential qualities derive from the ability of *Y. enterocolitica* to ferment mannitol conferring a deep red center to the flat yersinial colonies. Schiemann showed that this medium was of great value in discerning 63 *Y. enterocolitica* and *Y. enterocolitica*-like isolates which traversed the DNA homology groups of Brenner (15).

Soltesz and colleagues (49b) incorporated sodium oxalate into their so-called "Y" medium consisting of casein hydrolysate, peptone, bile salts, and lactose, and thereby formulated a selective and differential medium for the recovery of *Y. enterocolitica*. Using artificially infected stool specimens, these investigators reported superior isolation (99%) of *Y. enterocolitica* on the oxalate medium as compared (90%) to more standard media for recovery of *Y. enterocolitica* from clinical specimens. With the exception of desoxycholate agar, they did not include the more frequently used "enteric" media in their comparative studies.

Cold enrichment (4°C) of stool specimens in phosphate-buffered saline with weekly subculture for 28 days has been used to enhance recovery of *Y. enterocolitica* from fecal specimens (22,27,42,58,63). As noted in Table 6, this technique has been reported to yield *Y. enterocolitica* in the absence of isolation by conventional methods. From the data presented, however, cold enrichment appears of little value in the recovery of "classic" *Y. enterocolitica* serotypes (0:3, 0:5,27, 0:8, 0:9) from patients in the acute phase of gastroenteritis. When the organism is present in large numbers, it is readily isolated from culture media. In the convalescent phase, however, cold enrichment for 1-2 days does enhance recovery of *Y. enterocolitica* which may be shed in small numbers for up to four weeks after an acute episode of gastroenteritis (42). Pai and colleagues (42)

Table 6. Biotype and Serotype of *Yersinia enterocolitica* Isolated from Stools after Cold Enrichment

Author	Total	No. Isolated Routine	Cold(Days)	Biotype	Serotype(s)/no.	Author's Comment
Eiss Sweden (22)	49	34	15(5)	4 1 1	0:3(47) 0:5(1) 0:6(1)	Serotypes 0:3,0:8,0:9 grow well at 4°C, other serotypes more slowly.
Greenwood et al. USA (27)	1	0	1(21)	1	0:6	Short termed diarrhea in immuno-suppressed patient.
Pai et al. Canada (42)	181 27	147 7	34(1-21) 20(21)	4 3 2 1	0:3(181) 0:1,2,3,:0:2; 0:5(2); 0:5,27(4); 0:6,30(6): 0:6,31(2); 0:7,8(4),0:21; 0:34; nontypable (5);	Cold enrichment effective in asymptomatic and convalescent subjects - only minimally in patients with acute *Y. enterocolitica* 0:3 diarrhea. Clinical significance of the non-0:3 isolates uncertain.
Van Noyen et al. Belgium (58)	36	29	7(7-28)	4 1	0:3(29) 0:6;0:10;0:14 0:53; nontypable (3)	Biotype I isolates not recovered within 1 week of cold enrichment, repeat cultures negative. Serotypes 0:3,0:9 recovered 1 week. Agglutinins absent in serum of patients with biotype 1 isolates.
Weissfeld and Sonnenwirth USA (63)	6	0	6(7,14)	1	0:5(2);0:6,30: 0:7,8(2): nontyable	Patients with abdominal pain, diarrhea and fever, one with suspected obstruction - none found at surgery. Need for cold enrichment evident.

and van Noyen et al (58) have clearly shown that most *Y. enterocolitica* isolates recovered after prolonged cold enrichment (up to 28 days) are serologically heterogenous and generally biotype I strains (see below). With the exclusion of serotype 0:8 which is a biotype 1 organism, other biotype 1 isolates appear not to be human pathogens as they lack invasiveness and do not elicit an antibody response (1,2,31,55,58). While data support the non-pathogenicity of biotype 1 *Y. enterocolitica*, one must bear in mind that the acquisition of a plasmid coding for tissue invasiveness (65) would markedly alter the virulence potential of biotype 1 isolates, other than serotype 0:8. It would therefore seem prudent to assess each biotype 1 isolate for its virulence potential prior to concluding its etiologic significance. Alternatively, serum agglutinins against the isolate could also be assessed (11a).

Biochemically, with the exception of a group of selected tests, prior to the advent of ascribing species status to the diverse strains classified as *Y. enterocolitica*, there existed few reference points for definitive identification. These tests included negative reactions for oxidase, phenylalanine deaminase, lysine decarboxylase, arginine dihydrolase, and production of ornithine decarboxylase, urease, and B-galactosidase. While some isolates fermented sucrose and produced acetylmethylcarbinol others did not (*Y. kristensenii*); some were unable to utilize rhamnose while other isolates fermented this substrate rapidly especially at 25°C (*Y. intermedia*). It became apparent, therefore, that biochemical heterogeneity and temperature-influenced phenotypic characteristics both conspired to add a measure of confusion to *Y. enterocolitica*.

Presently, however, because of distinct species status accorded to "atypical" isolates, the biochemical identification and indeed speciation of yersiniae ensues in a logical fashion. While an occasional abberrant strain may be encountered such as a rapid lactose fermenter (18) or one that is urease negative (28), identification based on the features shown in Table 1 has been facilitated.

The relative biochemical variability among typical *Y. enterocolitica* isolates serves as a basis for "biotyping" isolates of human and environmental sources. Table 7 depicts the four schemes that have been utilized (4,30,39,61). It is stressed that the biotyping of *Y. enterocolitica* strains correlates well with the ecological, antigenic, and pathogenic attributes of this species. For instance, human pathogenic 0:3 isolates comprise biotype 4; 0:5 27 biotype 2; 0:8 biotype 1 (lecithinase positive, but salicin and esculin negative); and 0:9 biotype 2. It is important, however, to recognize that while the antigenic configuration of the classic human clinical isolates correlates well with biotyping, strains recovered from animal and environmental sources may possess 0 factors associated with human isolates. These, strains however are usually of a biotype not associated with their human-derived counterparts. Thus serotype 0:3 of biotype 1 and biochemically aberrant 0:8 strains have been isolated from nonhuman sources (M. Shayegani, New York State Department of Health).

II. EPIDEMIOLOGY

Epidemiologically, in the United States, there appears to be an ecological shift regarding the distribution of serotype 0:3 *Y. enterocolitica*. While this serotype is prevalent in Canada (phage type 9b) in Europe (phage type 8), and in South Africa (phage type 9A), as well as in other parts of the world, there has been a paucity of documentation of serotype 0:3 human infections in the United States. Of 29 *Y. enterocolitica* isolates submitted to the Center for Disease Control between 1966 and 1972, none were serotype 0:3 (62). In 1976, Bissett (5) reported the recovery of two serotype 0:3 isolates. In 1978 Thirumoorthi and Dajani (53) reported a patient who developed osteomyelitis of a rib caused by *Y. enterocolitica* serotype 0:3. In our own experience serving as an unofficial reference laboratory, 25 serotype 0:3 isolates have been

Table 7. Biotyping Schemata for *Y. enterocolitica*

	Y. entercolitica biotypes													
	Nilehn (39)					Wauters (61)					Knapp and Thal (30)			
Tests	1	2	3	4	5	1	2	3	4	5	1	2	3[a]	4[b]
Lecithinase	Not tested					+	0	0	0	0				
Salicin (acid)	+	0	0	0	0	Not tested					0	0	+	V
Esculin hydrolysis	+	0	0	0	0	Not tested					0	0	+	V
Indole production	+	+	0	0	0	+	+(L)	0	0	0	0	+	+	V
Xylose (acid)[c]	+	+	+	0	0	+	+	+	0	0	V	+	+	V
Lactose (acid, of medium)[c]	+	+	+	0	0	+	+	+	0	0				
Nitrate reduction	+	+	+	+	0	+	+	+	+	0				
Trehalose (acid)	+	+	+	+	0	+	+	+	+	0				
Sorbitol (acid)	+	+	+	+	0	Not tested								
Ornithine decarboxylase[c]	+	+	+	+	0	+	+	+	+	0				
Voges-Proskauer[c]	+	+	+	+	0	Not tested								
β-Galactosidase[c]	+	+	+	+	0	+	+	+	+	0				
Sucrose[c]	+	+	+	+	0	Not tested								
Sorbose	+	+	+	+	0	Not tested								

Bercovier (4)

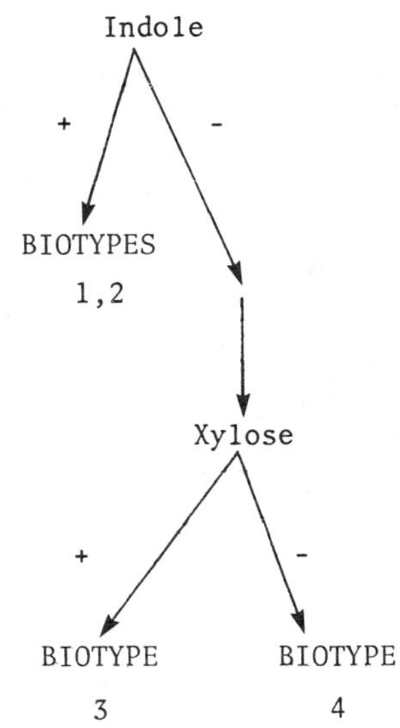

Note: OF, oxidation-fermentation; +, positive; 0, negative; V, variable.

[a]Strains in Group 3 may produce gas in glucose.

[b]Strains in Group 4 may show atypical reactions, i.e., lactose, rhamnose positive.

[c]Test performed at 25°C.

forwarded from hospitals in the surrounding New York City area and two additional isolates have been recovered in our laboratory (8a). These were recovered from patients without a travel history to endemic parts of the world. The incipient rise in serotype 0:3 isolates in the United States may reflect the establishment of a particular reservoir for this serotype within our geographical borders.

Conversely, while serotype 0:3 has appeared in the United States, the indigenous 0:8 serotype has not been recovered from environmental (water, milk, food products) or animal sources in other parts of the world. There is presently but a single human isolation reported in Europe (38a). Coupled to this enigma is the lack of isolation of serotype 0:9 outside of continental Europe (38).

Transmission of *Y. enterocolitica* from its natural reservoir to humans has been speculated to occur through inanimate sources such as water, contaminated foods or from another symptomatic (man, animal) subjects (26,36). The various temperature-related phenomena associated with virulence (invasiveness, enterotoxin production, intracellular survival) of *Y. enterocolitica*, and expressed only at lower temperatures, however, bespeak against the acquisition of the infecting strain from another "Hot" symptomatic host (7). Instead, it seems quite plausible that prior to human infection, the strain must pass from a "Hot" host through an inanimate "Cold" reservoir wherein it acquires its necessary surface components to colonize and invade the intestinal mucosa (Figure 5). Such a "Hot-Cold" cycle of transmission would even increase the inoculum densities of the infecting strain as *Y. enterocolitica* has been reported capable of multiplication at 4°C (22). Supporting this hypothesis are the reports of the Holland Patent outbreak which was traced to contaminated chocolate milk, and the typhoid-like bacteremia in a hunter (29). This latter subject fell ill during the winter while

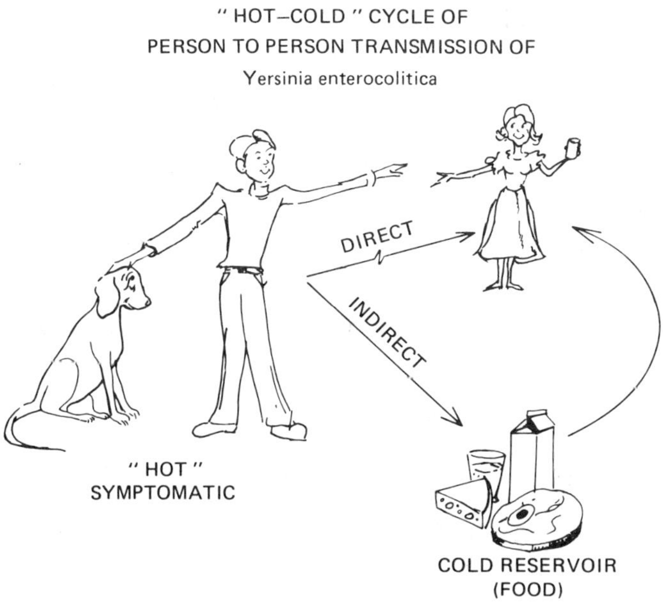

Fig. 5 In this schematic, transmission of *Yersinia enterocolitica* to another individual is postulated to occur after the microorganism has passed from a symptomatic subject through an inanimate (food, water) "cold" reservoir in which the necessary temperature-related virulence factors are acquired.

camping in the Adirondack Mountains of New York and drinking water from a stream from which a serotype 0:8 *Y. enterocolitica* was subsequently isolated.

III. PATHOGENESIS

Considering the pathogenesis of gastrointestinal *Y. enterocolitica* infections, one must be cognizant of aspects of the marked temperature-dependent expression of virulence factors such as tissue invasiveness and enterotoxin production.

Experimentally, using the rabbit and guinea pig models, it has been well documented that *Y. enterocolitica* and *Y. pseudotuberculosis* have the ability to penetrate the epithelial linings of intestinal mucosa as a prelude to establishing residence in their target reticuloendothelial tissue in the lamina propria and lymph follicles (54,56). In this regard, *Y. enterocolitica* and *Y. pseudotuberculosis* are place among the enteroinvasive intestinal pathogens such as *Salmonella, Shigella* and certain *Escherichia coli*. In contrast to the latter two species, however, yersiniae do not multiply within epithelial cells (19A).

Tissue invasiveness, as assessed by the elicitation of keratoconjunctivitis in Guinea pigs (Sereny Test) (49) or *in-vitro* in HeLa cells (Figure 6) has been elegantly demonstrated by Zink and

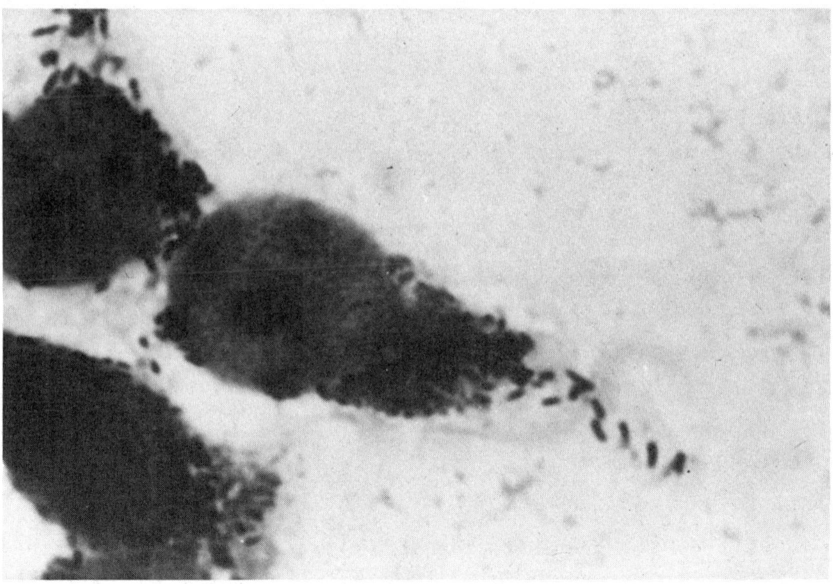

Fig. 6 HeLa cell invasion by *Yersinia enterocolitica* serotype 0:8 grown at 25°C. Note numerous bacillary forms within cytoplasm of infected cells. Experimental design after Lee et al. (31).

colleagues (65) to be a temperature-dependent plasmid-mediated function. These investigators correlated tissue invasiveness with the presence of a 41 × 10^6 MW plasmid harbored by the serotype O:8 strains tested (obtained during the Holland Patent outbreak). Three non O:8 isolates were noninvasive and lacked the 41 × 10^6 MW plasmid. Curing of O:8 strains with ethidium bromide resulted in loss of tissue invasiveness as did growth at 35°C. The study of Zink and co-workers defined a molecular mechanism to account for the earlier reports documenting loss of HeLa cell penetration by "classic" serotypes of *Y. enterocolitica* after cultivation at 37°C but not after 25°C incubation (55,58).

Following the studies of Zink and colleagues (65), Portnoy and co-workers (43a) showed that virulent strains of *Y. enterocolitica* possess a plasmid species ranging in mass from 40 to 48,000 MW. The presence of this class of plasmids could be associated with lethality for gerbils, but, however, not with tissue invasiveness. Strains which lost the 40-48 DNA plasmid species were still able to internalize in HEP-2 tissue culture cells. The 40-48 × 10^6 MW plasmid was, however, needed to induce detachment of the monolayer from the culture flask. Portnoy et al. postulated that tissue invasiveness may not be encoded for by plasmid DNA but rather that the plasmid-mediated determinants may be active after invasion. In this regard, the kerato-conjunctivitis (Sereny test) in Guinea pigs noted by Zink and colleagues (65) may actually be analogous to "monolayer detachment" which is associated with the presence of a class of plasmids in *Y. enterocolitica*.

It is of interest that although serotype O:3, O:5,27, O:8 and O:9 have been shown to invade HeLa cells (23,31,34a,43), serotype O:8 strains most consistently elicit a strong Sereny test (23,25, 38b,46b) defined by Schiemann and Devenish as guinea pig conjunctivitis (46b) (Table 8).

The events in the human host leading to either gastroenteritis as the major clinical presentation, or mesenteric adenitis or

Table 8. Correlation of Serotype and Biotype of *Yersinia enterocolitica* with Virulence Factors*

Serotype(s)	Biotype	ST[b]	Invasiveness HeLa**	Invasiveness Sereny**	VW Antigen
0:3	4	+	+	+0, weak +	+
0:5,27	2	+	+	0, weak +	+
0:6,30	1	+	+, weak	0, weak +	?
0:8	1	+	+	+	+
0:9	3	+	+	0	+
0:1; 0:1,2,3; 0:2,3; 0:4,32; 0:21	3,5	+	+	+	+
0:15a; 0:18; 0:20; 0:22	2	+(?)	+	0	?
Others[a]	1	+(10%)	0	0	?

*According to Feeley (23), Lee (31), Maki (34a), Mors (38a), Pai (41), Pedersen (43), Une (55), Schiemann and Devenish (46b,46c), Zink (65) and their colleagues.

**Temperature-dependent, + = positive, 0 = negative.

[a]Includes two sucrose negative isolates which were noninvasive. No data presented on enterotoxigenicity of these strains (43).

[b]ST = heat-stable enterotoxin.

terminal ileitis, (or combination of these features) are centrally focused upon tissue invasiveness, virulence of the individual strain, the ability of the host to contain the infection (age-related?) and the temporal relationship between the degree of symtomatology and the extent of intestinal involvement. As shown in Figure 7, following epithelial cell penetration of *Y. enterocolitica*, the microorganism passes into the lamina propria and muscularis mucosa. Depending upon inoculum densities (unknown), as well as the factors enumerated, during the first few weeks infection may be confined to the mucosa and result in an acute enteritis with abnormalities suggestive of superficial ulcerations (59). Occasionally, as revealed through autopsy studies (26), in protracted infection the

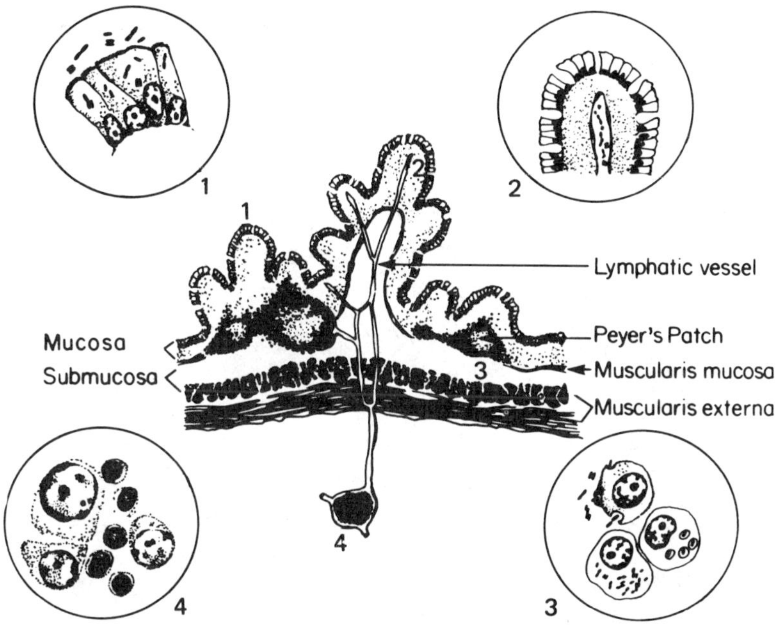

Fig. 7 Events in the pathogenesis of *Yersinia enterocolitica* enteric infection. 1. Adherence to and penetration of epithelial cells lining mucosa of bowel. 2,3. Passage of *Y. enterocolitica* through lamina propria to reticuloendothelial tissue in which multiplication takes place especially in Peyer's Patches which are abundent in terminal ileium. 4. Drainage of *Yersinia* through lymphatics to mesenteric lymph nodes resulting in inflammation, and occasionally ulceration of node. Drawings by Mei-Ku Huang, M.D.

entire gastrointestinal tract may show an ulcerative process, especially at the site(s) of increased mucosal lymphoid tissue. In children, gastroenteritis is the predominant clinical manifestation.

The second or concomitant presentation, as represented in Figure 7, is mesenteric lymphadenitis which occurs as a result of passage (extension) of the microorganism through the mucosa, submucosa, muscularis, and serosal layers with multiplication taking place within the reticuloendothelial (mononuclear) cells in the lamina propria and drainage to the mesenteric nodes via lymphatics. Inflamed and ulcerating lymph nodes account for the right iliac fossa syndrome simulating acute appendicitis (pseudoappendicitis). This syndrome is seldom seen in children less than five years of age although the ability to localize pain in this age group may be wanting. A case of pseudotumorigenic serotype 0:8 mesenteric lymphadenitis in a 2 month old child was recently published (3A).

Terminal ileitis results as a consequence of marked multiplication within the monomuclear cells of Peyer's patches which are especially abundant in the terminal ileum. Frequently, 10-20 mm of ileum will show ulcerations (59). In one post mortem finding approximately 1 meter of ileocaecum displayed a marked hemorrhagic necrosis and edema following serotype 0:3 infection (64).

In addition to tissue invasiveness and multiplication within reticuloendothelial cells, *Y. enterocolitica*, as well as 10% of rhamnose fermenting isolates tested (*Y. intermedia*?) (41) produce a heat stable enterotoxin active in suckling mice and the rabbit ileal loop. Enterotoxin synthesis is apparently chromosomally mediated (65) and the toxin is methanol soluble, acid stable (13), and its activity is similar to that of *E. coli* heat-stable enterotoxin (45). The role, however, of *Y. enterocolitica* enterotoxin in producing diarrheal manifestations is tempered by the fact that it is neither elaborated at 37°C growth temperatures (33,41) nor under anaerobiosis (45). Indeed, Schiemann has described an enterotoxin-negative strain of *Y. enterocolitica* serotype 0:3 which still produced diarrhea in experimentally infected mice (46a).

Recently, Carter and colleagues (16) and Gemski et al. (25) have shown that *Y. enterocolitica* serotype 0:8 possess in common with virulent *Y. pestis* and *Y. pseudotuberculosis* the V (protein) and W (lipoprotein) antigen complex. These antigenic determinants which are only produced at 37°C, are essential virulence factors (resistance to phagocytosis and to intracellular killing) of the plague bacillus. In *Y. enterocolitica*, by inference, it is thought that the V antigen is plasmid (VWA) coded and related to invasiveness since V+ strains are invasive and enterotoxigenic. Strains lacking WV antigen complex are noninvasive but still enterotoxigenic. These data support the findings of Zink et al. (35) regarding plasmid-mediated tissue invasiveness. The presence of the VWA plasmid in other *Yersinia* serotypes e.g., 0:3, 0:5,27, 0:9 remains to be demonstrated.

Analogous to the plague bacillus, *Y. pestis*, strains of *Y. enterocolitica* producing the VW antigen have a calcium dependency for growth at 37°C, but not at 25°C. Gemski and colleagues (25) showed that VW-positive strains could easily be differentiated from VW-negative strains by use of magnesium oxalate agar. On this medium, growth of VW-positive, invasive *Y. enterocolitica* is inhibited at 37°C but not at 25°C (VW antigen not synthesized at lower temperature). By way of contrast, isolates of *Y. enterocolitica* lacking the 42 × 10 MW plasmid associated with invasiveness which are hence VW-negative, lose their calcium dependency and readily grow on the magnesium oxalate agar at 37°C.

The magnesium oxalate agar inhibition test as applied to *Y. enterocolitica* by Gemski and colleagues (25) for distinguishing virulent from avirulent strains has been amplified to include testing of clinical isolates by Schiemann and colleagues (46c). These investigators coupled assays for calcium dependency at 35°C with the innovative autoagglutination in tissue culture assay developed by Laird and Cavanaugh (30a) for differentiating virulent from avirulent isolates. On the basis of these two parameters as well as the guinea pig conjunctivitis and mouse diarrhea models, Schiemann and co-workers showed that serotypes 0:3, 0:5,27, 0:8, 0:9, 0:4,32, and 0:21 were virulent. These isolates were, in addition, uniformly negative in esculin, salicin, rhamnose, and citrate reactions. As autoagglutination in tissue culture, and the production of the VW antigen are both temperature dependent, Laird and Cavanaugh suggest that autoagglutination may be an indicator of the determinant for VW positivity (30a). Virulence factors for *Y. enterocolitica* and methods for their assessment are listed in Table 9.

Table 9. Virulence Factors of *Yersinia Enterocolitica* and Methods for Their Assessment

Characteristic	Plasmid Associated	Method	Representative Serotypes	Comment
Adherence	?	Epithelial cell invasion	0:3	Temperature-dependent, (+) 25°C. Motility not a virulence factor.
Tissue Invasiveness	Lethality-yes Invasiveness?	HeLa, HEp-2 cell invasion Sereny test (10^{10} calls/ml).	0:3, 0:5,27 0:8, 0:9	HeLa cell invasion - lack of intracellular multiplication. Internalization process absence of 40-48 Mdal plasmid DNA.
		Pathogenicity for gerbils, mice.	0:8	
V-(protein)- W (Lipoprotein)	Yes	Growth of plasmid + strains inhibited on magnesium oxalate agar at 37°C, but not 25°C. Show calcium dependent growth at 37°C for expression of plasmid-associated properties.	0:8	Produced at 37°C only. Resist phagocytic killing, enhances survival within the reticuloendothelial system of host.
		Autoagglutination	0:3, 0:5,27 0:8, 0:9 0:4,32, 0:21	Temperature-dependent. May correlate with presence of VW antigen complex.

Clinically, other manifestations of *Y. enterocolitica* infection include the infrequently occurring acute typhoid-like septicemia or septicemia in compromised hosts (36), visceral (44) and superficial abscesses (34), and the postinfection sequelae of arthritis, erythema nodosum, glomerulonephritis, and myocarditis, occurring especially in patients in Scandinavian countries (32,33).

Temporally, we have seen that *Y. enterocolitica* has emerged as a multifaceted human pathogen. While the last decade has brought us to the brink of knowledge regarding numerous facets of the basic biology of this enigmatic microorganism, there still remain aspects in need of dissection.

As one envisions the subject of this report draped across the "microbiological horizon" (Figure 8) thoughts regarding factors accounting for the apparent restricted geographic distribution of "classic" serotypes of *Y. enterocolitica* are interwoven with those concerning the future role of environmental strains in human pathology (8).

In the United States we are apparently witnessing an ecological shift toward the establishment of a reservoir (animate? inanimate?) for serotype 0:3 phage type 9b strains (8a). Yet, serotype 0:9 has not been recorded as a causative agent of yersiniosis in the United States. Conversely, the "American" serotype 0:8 has apparently not caused widespread yersiniosis on a global basis.

Counterpointed against the geographic distribution of the classic pathogens is the tenuous role of the ubiquitous environmental strains in human disease. While these geographically, biochemically and serologically diverse strains lack enteroinvasiveness, their discountance as human pathogens is tempered by the feasibility of plasmid acquisition either from "classic" *Y. enterocolitica* or other *Enterobacteriaceae* engendering host-specific virulence factors. The public health significance of these species, mainly *Y. frederiksenii* and *Y. intermedia* in food products from which they have been recovered (31a) remains to be elucidated.

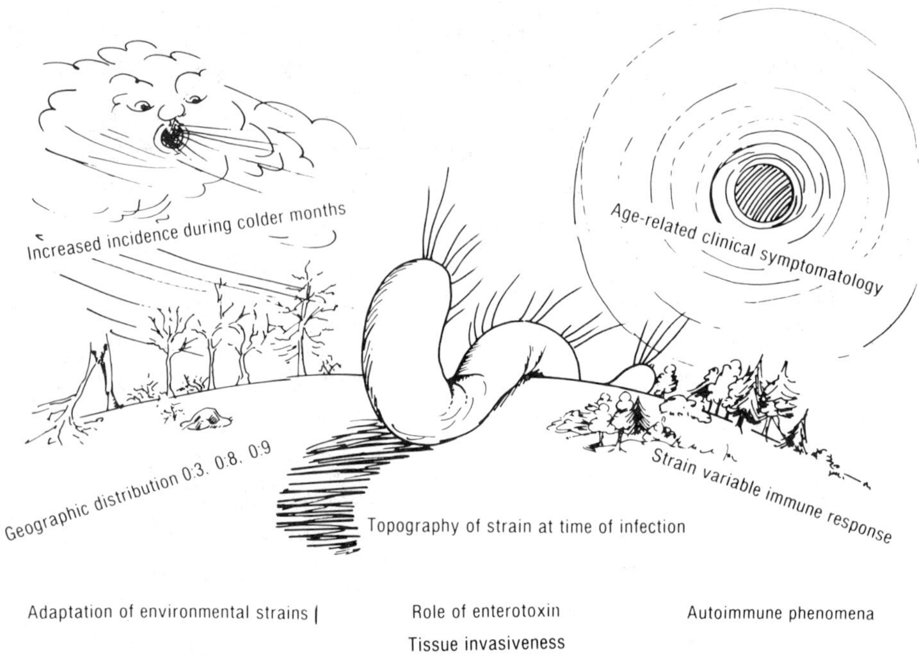

Fig. 8 *Yersinia enterocolitica* on imaginary "Microbiological Horizon" simultaneously inviting and defying total elucidation of the indicated intrinsic biologic phenomena.

Awaiting clarification is the nature of the surface topography of the infecting strain at the moment of acquisition and the series of events that ensue shortly after host and microbe interface. Such data is especially relevant as virulence factors such as tissue invasivness, intracellular survival, and enterotoxin production are temperature-sensitive and not expressed at body temperature. In this regard, does *Y. enterocolitica* undergo a "sheeding" of its outer surface after temperature adaptation in the human host? If so, what then is the contribution to pathogenesis of the VW antigen, expressed at 37°C? Does an "uncoating" of surface antigens acquired through the "cold" cycle permit adherence and tissue invasiveness and then give way to VW antigen which is protective? Support for such a hypothesis may be derived from the observation (E. Bottone, unpublished data) in two instances of the serum of patients agglutinating their own isolates to a greater titer after growth of the infecting strain at 25°C as compared to 37°C. This would suggest an important role for surface antigens in the initial host-microbe interaction.

Outstanding among the biologic nuances associated with *Y. enterocolitica* and seen mainly in patients in Europe, are the autoimmune phenomena. Questions as to incidence, mode of diagnosis, pathogenesis, genetic predisposition (HLA-B27 specificity), and demographic features all need further clarification. The concept of an "arthritogenic" strain of *Y. enterocolitica* (serotype O:3 phage type 8) enunciated by Ahvonen and Rossi (2a) and apparently non-existent in other parts of the world (20) is indeed intriguing. Equally tantalizing and without total explanation is the phenomenon of cross-reacting antibodies to *Y. enterocolitica* in the sera of patients with various thyroid disorders (49a).

It is apparent from the preceeding that the interest, fascination, and stimulation associated with the unraveling of the numerous facets of *Y. enterocolitica* will serve to ensure future research.

REFERENCES

1. Ahvonen, P. 1972. Human yersiniosis in Finland. I. Bacteriology and serology. Ann. Clin. Res. 4:30-38.

2. Ahvonen, P. 1972. Human yersiniosis in Finland. II. Clinical features. Ann. Clin. Res. 4:39-48.

2a. Ahvonen, P. and T. Rossi. 1970. Familial occurrence of *Yersinia enterocolitica* infection and acute arthritis. Acta Paediatr. Scand. Suppl. 206:121-122.

3. Alonso, J. M., J. Bejat, H. Bercovier, et H. Y. Mollaret. 1975. Sur un group de souches de *Yersinia enterocolitica* fermentant le rhamnose. Med. Mal. Infect. 10:490-492.

3a. Barlow, B., and R. Gandhi. 1981. Suppurative mesenteric adenitis: *Yersinia enterocolitica*. Amer. J. Dis. Child. 135: 171-172.

4. Bercovier, H., J. M. Alonso, Z. N. Bentaiba, and H. H. Mollaret. 1979. Contribution to the definition and the taxonomy of *Yersinia enterocolitica*. Contr. Microbiol. Immunol., P. B. Carter, L. Lafleur, and S. Toma (eds), 5:12-22, S. Karger, Basel.

4a. Bercovier, H., J. Ursing, D. J. Brenner, A. G. Steigerwalt, G. R. Fanning, G. P. Carter, and H. H. Mollaret. 1980. *Yersinia kristensenii*: a new species of *Enterobacteriaceae* composed of sucrose-negative strains (formerly called atypical *Yersinia enterocolitica* or *Yersinia enterocolitica*-like). Curr. Microbiol. 4:219-224.

5. Bissett, M. L. 1976. *Yersinia enterocolitica* isolates from humans in California. J. Clin. Microbiol. 4:137-144.

6. Black, R. E., R. J. Jackson, T. Tasi, M. Medevesky, M. Shayegani, J. C. Feeley, K. I. E. MacLeod, and A. M. Wakelee. 1978. Epidemic *Yersinia enterocolitica* infection due to contaminated chocolate milk. New Eng. J. Med. 298:76-79.

7. Bottone, E. J. 1977. *Yersinia enterocolitica*: A panoramic view of a charismatic microorganism. Crit. Rev. Microbiol. 5:211-241.

8. Bottone, E. J. 1978. Atypical *Yersinia enterocolitica*: Clinical and epidemiological parameters. J. Clin. Microbiol. 7:562-567.

8a. Bottone, E. J. 1983. Current trends of *Yersinia enterocolitica* isolates in the New York City area. J. Clin. Microbiol. 17:63-67.

9. Bottone, E. J., B. Chester, M. S. Malowany, and J. Allerhand. 1974. Unusual *Yersinia enterocolitica* isolates not associated with mesenteric lymphadenitis. Appl. Microbiol. 5:858-861.

10. Bottone, E. J., and T. Robin. 1977. *Yersinia enterocolitica:* Recovery and characterization of two unusual isolates from a case of acute enteritis. J. Clin. Microbiol. 5:341-345.

11. Bottone, E. J., K. Sandhu, and M. A. Pisano. 1980. *Yersinia intermedia:* Temperature-dependent bacteriocin production. J. Clin. Microbiol. 10:433-436.

11a. Bottone, E. J., and D. J. Sheehan. 1983. *Yersinia enterocolitica:* Guidelines for serologic diagnosis of human infections. Rev. Infect. Dis., Vol. 5, no. 5, Sept. - Oct.

12. Bowen, J. H., and S. D. Kominos. 1979. Evaluation of pectin agar medium for isolation of *Yersinia enterocolitica* within 48 hours. Amer. J. Clin. Pathol. 72:586-590.

13. Boyce, J. M., D. J. Evans, D. G. Evans, and H. L. DuPont. 1979. Production of heat-stable, methanol-soluble enterotoxin by *Yersinia enterocolitica*. Infect. Immun. 25:532-537.

14. Brenner, D. J. 1979. Speciation in *Yersinia*. Contr. Microbiol. Immunol., P. B. Carter, L. Lafleur, and S. Toma (eds.) 5:33-36, S. Karger, Basel.

14a. Brenner, D. J., H. Bercovier, J. Ursing, J. M. Alonso, A. G. Steigerwalt, G. R. Fanning, G. P. Carter, and H. H. Mollaret. 1980. *Yersinia intermedia:* a new species of *Enterobacteriaceae* composed of rhamnose-positive, melibiose-positive strains (formerly called *Yersinia enterocolitica* or *Yersinia enterocolitica*-like). Curr. Microbiol. 4:207-212.

15. Brenner, D. J., A. G. Steigerwalt, D. P. Falcao, R. E. Weaver, and G. R. Fanning. 1976. Characterization of *Yersinia enterocolitica* and *Yersinia pseudotuberculosis* by deoxyribonucleic acid hybridization and by biochemical reactions. Int. J. Syst. Bacteriol. 26:180-194.

16. Carter, P. B., R. J. Zahorchak, and R. R. Brubaker. 1980. Plague virulence antigens from *Yersinia enterocolitica*. Infect. Immun. 28:638-640.

17. Chester, B., G. Stotzky, E. J. Bottone, M. S. Malowany, and J. Allerhand. 1977. *Yersinia enterocolitica:* Biochemical, serological, and gas-liquid chromatographic characterization of rhamnose, raffinose, melibiose, and citrate utilizing strains. J. Clin. Microbiol. 6:461-468.

18. Cornelis, G., R. K. J. Luke, and M. H. Richmond. 1978. Fermentation of raffinose by lactose-fermenting strains of *Yersinia enterocolitica* and by sucrose-fermenting strains of *Escherichia coli*. J. Clin. Microbiol. 7:180-183.

19. Daniels, J. J. H. M., and C. Goudzwaard. 1963. Enkele stammern van een op *Pasteurella pseudotuberculosis* gelijkend niet geidentificiered species, geisoleerd bij knaagdieren. Tijdschrift voor Diergeneeskunde 88:96-102.

19a. Devenish, J. A., and D. A. Schiemann. 1981. HeLa cell infection by *Yersinia enterocolitica:* evidence for lack of intracellular multiplication and development of a new procedure for quantitative expression of infectivity. Infect. Immun. 32: 48-55.

20. Dickinson, A. B., and G. Mocquot. 1961. Studies on the bacterial flora of the alimentary tract of pigs, I. *Enterobacteriaceae* and other gram-negative bacteria. J. Appl. Bacteriol. 24:252-284.

21. Dudley, M. V. and E. B. Shotts, Jr. 1979. Medium for isolation of *Yersinia enterocolitica*. J. Clin. Microbiol. 10:180-183.

22. Eiss, J. 1975. Selective culturing of *Yersinia enterocolitica* at a low temperature. Scand. J. Infect. Dis. 7:249-251.

23. Feeley, J. C., J. G. Wells, T. F. Tsai, and N. D. Puhr. 1979. Detection of enterotoxigenic and invasive strains of *Yersinia enterocolitica*. Cont. Microbiol. Immunol., P. B. Carter, L. Lafleur, and S. Toma (eds.) 5:329-334, S. Karger, Basel.

24. Frederiksen, W. 1964. A study of some *Yersinia pseudotuberculosis*-like bacteria ("*Bacterium enterocoliticum*" and "*Pasteurella X*"). Proceedings of the XIV Scandinavian Congress of Pathology and Microbiology, pp. 103-104, Oslo.

25. Gemski, P., J. R. Lazere, and T. Casey. 1980. Plasmid associated with pathogenicity and cabcium dependency of *Yersinia enterocolitica*. Infect. Immun. 27:682-685.

26. Gutman, L. T., E. A. Ottesen, T. J. Quan, P. S. Noce, and S. L. Katz. 1973. An interfamilial outbreak of *Yersinia enterocolitica* enteritis. New Eng. J. Med. 288:1372-1377.

27. Greenwood, J. R., S. M. Flanigan, M. J. Pickett, and W. J. Martin. 1975. Clinical isolation of *Yersinia enterocolitica*: cold temperature enrichment. J. Clin. Microbiol. 2:559-560.

28. Housner, O. and S. H. Housenerova. 1979. The isolation of urease negative strains of *Yersinia enterocolitica*. Contr. Microbiol. Immunol., P. B. Carter, L. Lafleur, and S. Toma (eds.) 5:80-82, S. Karger, Basel.

29. Keet, E. E. 1974. *Yersinia enterocolitica* septicemia. Source of infection and incubation period identified. New York State J. Med. 74:2226-2230.

30. Knapp, W., and E. Thal. 1973. Differentiation of *Yersinia enterocolitica* by biochemical reactions. Contr. Microbiol. Immunol., S. Winblad (ed.), 2:10-15, S. Karger, Basel.

30a. Laird, W. J. and D. C. Cavanaugh. 1980. Correlation of autoagglutination and virulence in yersiniae. J. Clin. Microbiol. 11:430-432.

31. Lee, W. H., P. P. McGrath, P. H. Carter, and E. K. Eide. 1977. The ability of some *Yersinia enterocolitica* strains to invade HeLa cells. Can. J. of Microbiol. 23:1714-1722. 714-1722.

31a. Lee, W. H. 1977. An assessment of *Yersinia enterocolitica* and its presence in foods. J. of Food Protection 40:486-489.

32. Leino, R., and J. K. Kalliomaki. 1974. Yersiniosis as an internal disease. Ann. Int. Med. 81:458-461.

33. Lerisalo, M. 1978. Human *Yersinia enterocolitica* infections (Editorial). Ann. Clin. Res. 10:63-65.

34. Lewis, J. F., and J. Alexander. 1976. Facial abscess due to *Yersinia enterocolitica*. Am. J. Clin. Pathol. 66:1016-1018.

34a. Maki, M., P. Gronross, and T. Vesikari. 1978. In vitro invasiveness of *Yersinia enterocolitica* isolated from children with diarrhea. J. Infect. Dis. 138:677-680.

35. Malassez, L. and W. Vignal. 1883. Tuberculose zoogloeique (forme ou espece de tuberculose sans bacilles). Archives de Physiologie. Normale et Pathologique, 3 series, 2:369-412.

36. Mollaret, H. H. 1972. *Yersinia enterocolitica* infection. A new problem in pathology. Editorial Translation. Annales de Biologie Clinique, 30:1-6.

37. Mollaret, H. H. and P. Destombes. 1964. Les germes "X" en pathologic humaine. Presse Medicale 72:2913-2915.

38. Mollaret, H. H., H. Bercovier, and J. M. Alonso. 1979. Summary of the data received at the WHO Reference Center for *Yersinia enterocolitica*. Contr. Microbiol. Immunol. P. B. Carter, L. Lafleur, and S. Toma (eds.), 5:174-184, S. Karger, Basel.

38a. Monno, R., L. Marcuccio, I. Munno, G. Miragliotta, O. Brandonisio, D. Fumarola, and M. Montinari. 1981. Prima segnalazione in Puglia di isolamento di *Yersinia enterocolitica* in compo pediatrico. Ann. Sclavo. 23:87-91.

38b. Mors, V., and C. H. Pai. 1980. Pathogenic properties of *Yersinia enterocolitica*. Infect. Immun. 28:292-294.

39. Nilehn, B. 1969. Studies on *Yersinia enterocolitica*. Acta Pathol. Microbiol. Scand. 206:1-48.

40. Nilehn, B. 1973. The relationship of incubation temperature to serum bactericidal effect, pathogenicity and *in vivo* survival of *Yersinia enterocolitica*. In: Contr. Microbiol. Immunol., S. Winblad (ed.), 2:85-92, S. Karger, Basel.

41. Pai, C. H., and V. Mors. 1978. Production of enterotoxin by *Yersinia enterocolitica*. Infect. Immun. 19:908-911.

42. Pai, C. H., S. Sorger, L. Lafleur, L. Lackman, and M. Marks. 1979. Efficacy of cold enrichment techniques for recovery of *Yersinia enterocolitica* from human stools. J. Clin. Microbiol. 9:712-715.

43. Pedersen, K. B., S. Winblad, and V. Bitsch. 1979. Studies on the interaction between different O-serotypes of *Yersinia enterocolitica* and HeLa cells. Acta. Path. Microbiol. Scand. Sect. B. 87:141-145.

43a. Portnoy, D. A., S. L. Moseley, and S. Falkow. 1981. Characterization of plasmids and plasmid-associated determinants of *Yersinis enterocolitica* pathogenesis. Inf. Immun. 31:779-782.

44. Rabson, A. R., A. F. Hallett, and H. J. Koornhoff. 1975. Generalized *Yersinia enterocolitica* infection. J. Infect. Dis. 131:447-451.

45. Robins-Browne, R. M., C. S. Still, M. D. Miliotis, and H. J. Koornhof. 1979. Mechanism of action of *Yersinia enterocolitica* enterotoxin. Infect. Immunol. 25:680-684.

46. Schiemann, D. A. 1979. Synthesis of selective agar medium for isolation of *Yersinia enterocolitica*. Can. J. Microbiol. 25:1298-1304.

46a. Schiemann, D. A. 1981. An enterotoxin-negative strain of *Yersinia enterocolitica* serotype 0:3 is capable of producing diarrhea in mice. Inf. Immun. 32:571-574.

46b. Schiemann, D. A., and J. A. Devenish. 1980. Virulence of *Yersinia enterocolitica* determined by lethality in Mongolian gerbils and by the Sereny test. Infect. Immum. 29:500-506.

46c. Schiemann, D. A., J. A. Devenish, and S. Toma. 1981. Characteristics of virulence in human isolates of *Yersinia enterocolitica*. Infect. Immun. 32:400-403.

46d. Schiemann, D. A., and J. A. Devenish. 1982. Relationship of HeLa cell infectivity to biochemical, serological, and virulence characteristics of *Yersinia enterocolitica*. Infect. Immun. 35:497-506.

47. Schleifstein, J., and M. B. Coleman. 1939. An unidentified microorganism resembling *A. lignieri* and *Past. pseudotuberculosis* and pathogenic for man. New York State J. Med. 39:1749-1753.

48. Schleifstein, J., and M. Coleman. 1943. *Bacterium enterocoliticum*. Annual Report of the Division of Laboratories and Research, p. 56. New York State Department of Health.

49. Sereny, B. 1955. Experimental *Shigella keratoconjunctivitis*. A preliminary report. Acta. Microbiol. Acad. Sci. Hung. 2:293-296.

49a. Shenkman, L., and E. J. Bottone. 1976. Antibodies to *Yersinia enterocolitica* in thyroid disease. Ann. Int. Med. 85:735-739.

49b. Soltesz, L. V., C. Schalen, and P. Mardh. 1980. An effective, selective medium for *Yersinia enterocolitica* containing sodium oxalate. Acta Path. Microbiol. Scand. 88:11-16.

50. Sonnenwirth, A. C. 1970. Bacteremia with and without meningitis due to *Yersinia enterocolitica, Edwardsiella tarda, Commamonas terrigena* and *Pseudomonas maltophilia*. Ann. New York Acad. Sci. 174:488-502.

51. Sonnenwirth, A. C. and R. E. Weaver. 1970. *Yersinia enterocolitica* (Letter to Editor). New Eng. J. Med. 283:1468.

52. Thal, E. 1954. Untersuchungen uber *Pasteurella pseudotuberkulosis*. Thesis Berlingska Boktryckeriet, Lund.

53. Thirumoorthi, M., and A. S. Dajani. 1978. *Yersinia enterocolitica* osteomyelitis in a child. Amer. J. Dis. Child. 132: 578-580.

54. Une, T. 1977. Studies on the pathogenicity of *Yersinia enterocolitica* I. Experimental infection in rabbits. Microbiol. Immunol. 21:349-363.

55. Une, T. 1977. Studies on the pathogenicity of *Yersinia enterocolitica* II. Interaction with cultured cells in vitro. Microbiol. and Immunol. 21:365-377.

56. Une, T. 1977. Studies on the pathogenicity of *Yersinia enterocolitica* III. Comparative studies between *Y. enterocolitica* and *Y. pseudotuberculosis*. Microbiol. and Immunol. 21:505-516.

56a. Ursing, J., D. J. Brenner, H. Bercovier, G. R. Fanning, A. G. Steigerwalt, J. Brault, and H. H. Mollaret. 1980. *Yersinia frederiksenii:* a new species of *Enterobacteriaceae* composed of rhamnose-positive strains (formerly called atypical *Yersinia enterocolitica* or *Yersinia enterocolitica*-like). Curr. Microbiol. 4:213-217.

57. Van Loghem, J. J. 1944. The classification of the plague bacillus. J. Microbiol. and Serol. 10:15-16.

58. Van Noyen, R., J. Vandepitte, and G. Wauters. 1980. Nonvalue of cold enrichment of stools for isolation of *Yersinia enterocolitica* serotypes 3 and 9 from patients. J. Clin. Microbiol. 11:127-131.

59. Vantroppen, G., H. O. Agg, E. Ponette, K. GeBoes, and P. H. Bertrand. 1977. *Yersinia* enteritis and enterocolitis: gastroenterological aspects. Gastroenterol. 72:220-227.

60. Von Riesen, V. L. 1975. Polypectate digestion of *Yersinia*. J. Clin. Microbiol. 2:552-553.

61. Wauters, G. 1970. Contribution a l'etude de *Yersinia enterocolitica*. These d'agrege University Catholique de Louvain, Vander, London.

62. Weaver, R. E., and J. G. Jordan. 1973. Recent human isolates of *Yersinia enterocolitica* in the United States. Contr. Microbiol. and Immunol., S. Winblad (ed.), 2:120-125, S. Karger, Basel.

63. Weissfeld, A. S., and A. C. Sonnenwirth. 1980. *Yersinia enterocolitica* in adults with gastrointestinal disturbances: need for cold enrichment. J. Clin. Microbiol. 11:196-197.

64. Zen-Yoji, H., and T. Maruyama. 1972. The first successful isolations and identification of *Yersinia enterocolitica* from human cases in Japan. Jap. J. Microbiol. 16:493-500.

65. Zink, D. L., J. C. Feeley, J. G. Wells, C. Vanderzant, J. C. Vickery, W. D. Roof, and G. A. O'Donovan. 1980. Plasmid-mediated tissue invasiveness in *Yersinia enterocolitica*. Nature 283:224-226.

3

Noncholera *Vibrio* Gastroenteritis

DON J. BRENNER
Division of Bacterial Diseases
Center for Infectious Diseases
Centers for Disease Control
Atlanta, Georgia

Until quite recently (and still, in the minds of many), the species *Vibrio cholerae* was considered by most epidemiologists and many clinical bacteriologists to consist only of the epidemic serotype, 01. The terms nonagglutinating *Vibrio* (NAG) or noncholera *Vibrio* (NCV) were used to describe any organism that was culturally or biochemically similar to *V. cholerae* 01 but did not agglutinate with 01 antiserum. Included under the NAG and NCV umbrella were all *V. cholerae* serotypes other than 01, other *Vibrio* species, *Aeromonas* species, and *Plesiomonas shigelloides*.

NAG, even when restricted to *Vibrio* species or to strains of *V. cholerae* other than 01, is a misleading and an incorrect term.

These organisms possess 0 antigens and are perfectly capable of agglutinating. They just do not agglutinate with 01 antiserum because they do not have the 01 antigen. There are at least 100 known 0 antigen groups in *Vibrio cholerae* (22,23,25,27).

NCV is also both a misleading and an incorrect designation. In the first place, data from throughout the world indicate that *V. cholerae* serotypes other than 01 can cause cholera -- from a mild form of disease to cholera gravis (severe cases) which can certainly be fatal. The only etiologic difference is that the non-01 strains cause sporadic cases and an occasional limited epidemic, whereas only 01 strains are responsible for large-scale epidemics and pandemics. The reason for this difference is unknown.

Quarantine regulations are specifically written around *V. cholerae* serotype 01, because of its international public health importance. Nonetheless, a patient suffering from full-blown rice-stool diarrhea caused by a non-01 serotype will not be impressed if told he does not have cholera. Furthermore, regardless of clinical importance, differences in virulence, pathogenicity or infectivity are not a sufficient basis for speciation. All serotypes of bacteria that are biochemically (13) and genetically (7) similar to *V. cholerae* are in fact, *V. cholerae* -- just as all serotypes of *Escherichia coli*, whether pathogenic or not, are *E. coli*.

It is confusing and essentially meaningless to categorize other vibrios, *Aeromonas* and *Plesiomonas* as noncholera vibrios. Since NAG or NCV is usually not defined in the literature, their meaning is unclear. These terms (the title of this presentation not withstanding) should not be used. The distinction used at the Centers for Disease Control (CDC) is *V. cholerae* 01 and *V. cholerae* non-01 (or non-01 *V. cholerae*). At CDC we explain these designations as follows:

> *V. cholerae* 01. This is the epidemic serotype. Each case should be immediately reported to the appropriate public health officials in your institution and your State health laboratory.

V. cholerae Smith type 17 (CDC uses the O antigen typing system of H. L. Smith [27]). This is not the epidemic strain of *V. cholerae*. CDC recommends that each case be investigated to ascertain the mode of transmission. Assistance can be obtained through your State Health Laboratory and Epidemiologist and, through them, from CDC.

Vibrio cholerae is identified biochemically according to reactions described by Ewing, Davis, and Martin (8) and reprinted in several places, including the second edition of the Manual of Clinical Microbiology (9). All human isolates and environmental isolates of public health significance are serotyped. Three subserotypes of 01 exist. They are in an AB-AC-ABC relationship, in which A is common to all 01 strains. *V. cholerae* 01 strains may be further subdivided by Heiberg grouping (11), biotyping into classical or eltor biotypes (8), and phage typing (18), which has been updated by Lee and Furniss.

The final parameter tested in *V. cholerae* isolates is the ability to produce choleratoxin (CT). It is often assumed that there is a 1:1 correlation between the 01 serotype and CT production. This is not true. To my knowledge all strains of *V. cholerae* 01 isolated from symptomatic humans produced CT. Strains directly associated with human infection -- sewage near the home of a patient or food incriminated as the vehicle of infection -- are CT-positive. Thus far, all strains of *V. cholerae* 01 isolated from the environment in the absence of human infection are CT-negative. All environmental non-01 *V. cholerae* isolates are CT-negative. Most, but not all, human isolates of non-01 *V. cholerae* are also CT-negative. In summary, ALL ENVIRONMENTAL ISOLATES OF *V. cholerae*, regardless of serotype, are CT-negative. All human 01 isolates and some human non-01 isolates are CT-positive. Thus serotype, source of isolation presence of associated human cases, and the ability to product CT must be carefully weighed before attempting to define the public health significance of environmental isolates.

There were no indigenous cases of 01 cholera in the United States for the first 75 years of this century. In 1973 there was an isolate from a man in Texas and a second case occurred in Alabama in 1977. In 1978 a cluster of at least 11 cases of cholera caused by *V. cholerae* eltor 01 Inaba occurred in Louisiana. These cases were associated with the consumption of crabs and possibly shrimp (3). In 1980, a dozen or more cases of cholera were found in Laotian refugees. The states affected included California, Pennsylvania and Maryland. The causative organism was *V. cholerae* eltor 01 Ogawa.

Human isolates of non-01 *V. cholerae* from both intestinal and systemic infection have increased substantially throughout the 1970's. Much of this increase is undoubtedly due to improved culturing methods. Cases between 1972 and 1975 have been reviewed by Hughes et al. (14), who found that shellfish and exposure to salt water were the most common factors in non-01 infection. This trend is continuing, as judged by several recent cases in Florida where hunters who ate raw oysters contracted cholera.

Vibrio parahaemolyticus, Vibrio alginolyticus, Vibrio vulnificus, Vibrio fluvialis, Vibrio mimicus, Vibrio damsela, Vibrio hollisae, and *Vibrio metschnikovii* are also involved in human infection. If we extend our scope to the family *Vibrionaceae* (or to the scope of noncholera vibrios), we must also include *Aeromonas hydrophila* and *Plesiomonas shigelloides*.

V. parahaemolyticus is the leading cause of food poisoning in Japan, where the vehicle is most often raw fish. It is also a significant cause of sporadic and epidemic food poisoning in the United States, having been implicated in 14 outbreaks between 1971 and 1978 (2,6). In the continental United States *V. parahaemolyticus* food poisoning is caused by consuming cooked shellfish, especially crab and shrimp, or cooked fish, although an outbreak in Hawaii in 1972 was attributed to the consumption of raw crab (1). Thus, infection is most likely caused by undercooking, or improper handling after cooking. Wound infections obtained in a marine environment are occasionally caused by *V. parahaemolyticus* (2). The disease is usually characterized by watery diarrhea, abdominal cramps, nausea and vomiting. It has a mean duration of 3 days; no fatalities have been reported in the United States. A very high correlation has been obtained in Japan between the Kanagawa phenomenon (hemolysis on Wagatsuma agar) and gastroenteritis (21). More than 96% of *V. parahaemolyticus* isolates from stools of patients with diarrhea were Kanagawa-positive, whereas only 1% of environmental isolates were positive. This test is not used routinely in the United States so comparable data are unavailable. *V. parahaemolyticus* food poisoning occurs mainly between June and October (2).

Vibrio alginolyticus is isolated almost exclusively from wounds or ear infections associated with swimming or a marine environment (19,20). Although an occasional stool isolate has been recovered from patients with diarrhea, *V. alginolyticus* was not judged to be the etiologic agent.

Vibrio vulnificus, formerly referred to as lactose-positive, halophilic *Vibrio* or *"Beneckea vulnifica,"* was first isolated and characterized in the mid-1960's (12). The clinical characteristics of disease caused by *V. vulnificus* were recently reviewed by Blake et al. (4). Two types of disease have been characterized. One is a septicemia occurring after consumption of raw oysters. This disease is often found in patients with pre-existing liver disease, and fatality rates are high. Wound infections due to *V. vulnificus* are usually associated with injuries associated with handling crabs or with exposure to sea water.

Vibrio mimicus was formerly called a sucrose-negative *V. cholerae*. It has been isolated from shellfish and water, as well as from cases of human disease, including diarrhea and ear infections. In most human cases the consumption of raw shellfish was the suspected vehicle of infection (7a). Most *V. mimicus* strains are typable with antisera against *V. cholerae* and strains from 3 serogroups produced either a heat-labile or heat-stable enterotoxin (7a).

Vibrio damsela has been isolated from skin ulcers on a species of damselfish, and from at least seven human wound infections (16a).

Vibrio hollisae was isolated from 14 human stools, one small intestinal and one blood specimen. Several strains were isolated as pure cultures from stools of people with diarrhea. Raw seafood is again the suspected vehicle of infection (11a).

Vibrio metschnikovii has been isolated from the intestines of man and animals, as well as from many types of shellfish, sewage, rivers and estuaries (16). There is no published evidence that it causes disease, although an isolate from blood was received at CDC.

Vibrio fluvialis was described by Furniss et al. in England as group F (10) and was subsequently shown to be the same as the CDC group EF-6 (5). There are two biogroups which differ in the ability to produce gas from glucose. Both biogroups have been isolated from rivers, estuaries and shellfish in many parts of the world. Most human isolates are from Asia and Africa. *V. fluvialis* was isolated from many patients in a diarrheal outbreak affecting some 500 patients in Bangladesh (15). Although definitive studies have not been done, *V. fluvialis* must be considered as a potentially pathogenic organism.

Transport, culture, and isolation procedures for vibrios have been reviewed by Feeley and Balows (9). As for other causative agents of gastroenteritis, stool samples should be collected as soon as possible, certainly before the initiation of antibiotic therapy. When immediate culturing is not possible, Cary-Blair transport medium is recommended. Tellurite-taurocholate peptone broth has been successfully used as an enrichment-transport medium (17). Buffered glycerol saline is not a suitable transport medium for *Vibrio* species.

For isolation, specimens should be inoculated on a nonselective medium. Taurocholate gelatin agar is preferred, but nutrient agar is also suitable. Heavy inoculation is made on selective media, of which thiosulfate-citrate bile salts sucrose agar (TCBS) is by far the most popular. Tellurite-taurocholate gelatin agar may also be used as a selective medium for the isolation of *Vibrio* species. The preferred enrichment medium is tellurite-taurocholate alkaline broth. Alkaline peptone broth, pH 8.4 to 8.5, also can be used to enrich vibrios. Enrichment cultures should be incubated at 36 ± 1 C for 6 to 8 h (or, if impractical, overnight) and then subcultured to selective and nonselective media. It must be emphasized that *V. cholerae* and other *Vibrio* species grow poorly or not at all on media commonly used for *Enterobacteriaceae:* Salmonella-Shigella, eosin methylene blue, brilliant green, etc., although most strains grow on MacConkey agar.

The biochemical reactions used to identify *Vibrio* species are very similar to those used for *Enterobacteriaceae*. Additional tests that are important for *V. cholerae* are the string test (26) and sensitivity to the vibriostatic pteridine compound 0/129 (24).

The biochemical reactions of *Vibrio* species are given by the authors already cited. One major caveat is that several of these species cannot grow in the absence of salt. *V. cholerae* biochemical reactions are done with media prepared as for *Enterobacteriaceae*. In our laboratories carbohydrate base normally contains 0.5% NaCl, and this is not further supplemented. One percent NaCl is added to media that normally do not contain salt, such as indole, methyl red, Voges-Proskauer, decarboxylases, gelatin, nitrate and indophenol oxidase.

All *Vibrio* species are oxidase-positive (except *V. metschnikovii*) and bear monotrichous, polar flagella. Either of these characteristics is sufficient to separate them from all species in the family *Enterobacteriaceae*. *V. metschnikovii* is oxidase-negative and nitrate-negative, which separates it from all species in the family *Vibrionaceae*. Tests of value in differentiating *Vibrio* species are found in references 7a and 11a.

Vibrio cholerae and *V. parahaemolyticus* are present and are significant causes of gastrointestinal disease in the United States. We do not yet know the incidence or clinical relevance of *Vibrio fluvialis* or of *V. metschnikovii*. *V. vulnificus* and, to a lesser extent, *V. alginolyticus* are extraintestinal pathogens. Laboratories should use media on which these organisms can be isolated -- TCBS is the key -- and should be able to identify these organisms.

REFERENCES

1. Barker, W. H., Jr. 1974. *Vibrio parahaemolyticus* outbreaks in the United States. Lancet i:551-554.

2. Barker, W. H., R. E. Weaver, G. K. Morris, and W. T. Martin. 1974. Epidemiology of *Vibrio parahaemolyticus* infections in humans. In: Microbiology 1974, American Society for Microbiology, Washington, D.C., pp. 257-262.

3. Blake, P. A., D. T. Allegra, J. D. Snyder, T. J. Barrett, L. McFarland, C. T. Caraway, J. C. Feeley, J. P. Craig, J. V. Lee, N. D. Puhr, and R. A. Feldman. 1980. Cholera: a possible endemic focus in the United States. New England Journal of Medicine 302:305-309.

4. Blake, P. A., M. H. Merson, R. E. Weaver, D. G. Hollis, and P. C. Heublein. 1979. Disease caused by a marine *Vibrio*: clinical characteristics and epidemiology. New England Journal of Medicine 300:1-5.

5. Brenner, D. J., R. E. Weaver, D. G. Hollis, and B. R. Davis. 1979. The EF-6 group of *Vibrio*-like bacteria. Abstracts of the Annual Meeting of the American Society for Microbiology, p. 35.

6. Center for Disease Control. 1978. Morbidity and Mortality Weekly Report 27:345-346.

7. Citarella, R. V., and R. R. Colwell. 1970. Polyphasic taxonomy of the genus *Vibrio*: polynucleotide sequence relationships among selected *Vibrio* species. Journal of Bacteriology 104: 434-442.

7a. Davis, B. R., G. R. Fanning, J. M. Madden, A. G. Steigerwalt, H. B. Bradford, Jr., H. L. Smith, Jr., and D. J. Brenner. 1981. Characterization of biochemically atypical *Vibrio cholerae* strains and designation of a new pathogenic species, *Vibrio mimicus*. Journal of Clinical Microbiology 14:631-639.

8. Ewing, W. H., B. R. Davis, and W. J. Martin. 1966. Outlines of methods for the isolation and identification of *Vibrio cholerae*. Center for Disease Control, Atlanta, Georgia.

9. Feeley, J. C., and A. Balows. 1974. *Vibrio*. In: "Manual of Clinical Bacteriology," second edition, E. H. Lennette, E. H. Spaulding, and J. P. Truant, editors, American Society for Microbiology, Washington, D.C., pp. 238-245.

10. Furniss, A. L., J. V. Lee, and T. J. Donovan. 1977. Group F, a new vibrio? Lancet ii:565-566.

11. Heiberg, B. 1936. The biochemical reactions of vibrios. Journal of Hygiene (Cambridge) 36:114-117.

11a. Hickman, F. W., J. J. Farmer III, D. G. Hollis, G. R. Fanning, A. G. Steigerwalt, R. E. Weaver, and D. J. Brenner. 1982. Identification of *Vibrio hollisae* sp. nov. from patients with diarrhea. Journal of Clinical Microbiology 15:395-401.

12. Hollis, D. G., R. E. Weaver, C. N. Baker, and C. Thornsberry. 1976. A halophilic *Vibrio* species isolated from blood cultures. Journal of Clinical Microbiology 3:425-431.

13. Hugh, R., and R. Sakazaki. 1972. Minimal number of characters for the identification of *Vibrio* species, *Vibrio cholerae*, and *Vibrio parahaemolyticus*. Journal of the Conference of Public Health Laboratory Directors, 31:133-137.

14. Hughes, J. M., D. G. Hollis, E. J. Gangarosa, and R. E. Weaver. 1978. Non-cholera *Vibrio* infections in the United States. Annals of Internal Medicine 88:602-606.

15. Huq, I. M., M. U. Khan, K. M. S. Aziz, and D. J. Brenner. 1979. Studies on the newly recognized group of organisms termed EF-6, isolated from an unusual epidemic causing diarrhea. Abstracts, 15th Joint Conference on Cholera, U.S.-Japan Cooperative Medical Science Program, p. 68.

16. Lee, J. V., T. J. Donovan, and A. L. Furniss. 1978. Characterization, taxonomy, and emended description of *Vibrio metschnikovii*. International Journal of Systematic Bacteriology 28: 99-111.

16a. Love, M., D. Teebken-Fisher, J. E. Hose, J. J. Farmer III, F. W. Hickman, and G. R. Fanning. 1981. *Vibrio damsela*, a marine bacterium, causes skin ulcers on the damselfish *Chromis punctipinnus*. Science 214:1139-1140.

17. Monsur, K. A. 1963. Bacteriological diagnosis of cholera under field conditions. Bulletin of the World Health Organization 28:387-389.

18. Muckerjee, S., 1963. The bacteriophage susceptibility test in differentiating *Vibrio cholerae* and *Vibrio el tor*. Bulletin of the World Health Organization 28:333-336.

19. Pien, F., K. Lee, and H. Higa. 1977. *Vibrio alginolyticus* infections in Hawaii. Journal of Clinical Microbiology 5:672.

20. Rubin, S. J., and R. C. Tilton. 1975. Isolation of *Vibrio alginolyticus* from wound infections. Journal of Clinical Microbiology 2:556-558.

21. Sakazaki, R. 1979. *Vibrio* infections. In: "Food-borne Infections and Intoxications," second edition, Academic Press, New York, pp. 173-209.

22. Sakazaki, R., and T. Shimada. 1977. Report: serovars of *Vibrio cholerae* identified during 1970-1975. Japanese Journal of Medical Science and Biology 30:279-282.

23. Sakazaki, R., K. Tamura, C. Z. Gomez, and R. Sen. 1970. Serological studies on the cholera group of vibrios. Japanese Journal of Medical Science and Biology 23:13-20.

24. Shewan, J. M., W. Hodgkiss, and J. Liston. 1954. A method for the rapid differentiation of certain nonpathogenic, asporogenous bacilli. Nature (London) 173:208-209.

25. Shimada, T., and R. Sakazaki. 1977. Additional serovars and inter-O antigenic relationships of *Vibrio cholerae*. Japanese Journal of Medical Science and Biology 30:275-277.

26. Smith, H. L., Jr. 1970. A presumptive test for vibrios: the "string" test. Bulletin of the World Health Organization 42:817-818.

27. Smith, H. L., Jr. 1979. Serotyping of non-cholera vibrios. Journal of Clinical Microbiology 10:85-90.

4

Aeromonas and *Plesiomonas* as Agents of Diarrhea

ALEXANDER von GRAEVENITZ
Department of Medical Microbiology
University of Zurich
Zurich, Switzerland

Papers on the ecology and clinical significance of the genera *Aeromonas* and *Plesiomonas* have become rather numerous in the past decade. Some of them are quoted in the reference section of this paper, which covers only the relationship of these bacteria to enteric disease. Biochemical and taxonomic considerations are reviewed briefly for diagnostic reasons. More extensive reviews have been published elsewhere (39,46,69).

I. TAXONOMIC AND BIOCHEMICAL ASPECTS

The genera *Aeromonas* and *Plesiomonas* belong to the family *Vibrionaceae*. Its members are gram-negative, polarly flagellated, facultatively anaerobic, fermentative, oxidase-positive rods.

Members of the genus *Aeromonas* are usually montrichous, may or may not produce gas with glucose fermentation, do not decarboxylate ornithine, and form many exoenzymes like ribonuclease, deoxyribonuclease, elastase, phospholipase A and B, phosphatase, fibrinolysin, gelatinase, caseinase, and lipase (39). They are insensitive to the compound 0/129 (2,4-diamino-6,7-diisopropylpteridine) and have a guanine-cytosine (GC) ratio of 57-63 moles % (69). A still unresolved difficulty is the speciation of the genus. Schubert (56) has delineated the species *A. hydrophila* (with the subspecies *hydrophila, anaerogenes,* and *proteolytica*), *A. punctata* (with the ssp. *punctata* and *caviae*), and *A. salmonicida* (with the ssp. *salmonicida, achromogenes,* and *masoucida*). The species *A. salmonicida* as well as *A. hydrophila ssp. proteolytica* have only been found associated with cold-blooded animals. On the other hand, Popoff and Véron (45) have recognized three species: *A. hydrophila* (biovars *hydrophila* and *anaerogenes*), *A. sobria,* and *A. salmonicida* (for their biochemical reactions, see the original articles and a review (45,56,69)).

The genus *Plesiomonas* carries only one species, *P. shigelloides* (formerly A. shigelloides) (57), which is mainly lophotrichous, ferments fewer carbohydrates than *Aeromonas* (without gas formation), is ornithine and lysine positive, and forms no exoenzymes. The GC ratio is 51 mol %. Some strains share the 0 antigen with *Shigella sonnei* phase 1. It is 0/129 sensitive.

The most important differential characters between these genera and the various species of *Vibrio* recognized at this time are listed in Table 1. The most recently delineated species, *V. damsela* and *V. hollisae* (28a), are not listed. More comprehensive data can be found elsewhere (69).

A number of caveats apply.

1. So far, data bases of commercial kits do not include all *Vibrio* and *Aeromonas* species mentioned in Table 1 (16,52);
2. The oxidase test is usually reversed at pH $\leq$ 5.1 (30). If a sugar incorporated in the growth medium is fermented (e.g., lactose in MacConkey agar by *A. hydrophila*), a

Table 1. Most Important Tests in the Differential Diagnosis of Vibrionaceae

Test	V. cholerae	V. mimicus	V. vulnificus	V. fluvialis	V. metschnikovii	V. parahaemolyticus	V. alginolyticus	Aeromonas	Ples. shig.
Oxidase	+	+	+	+	-	+	+	+	+
DNase	+	+	+	+	+	+	+	+	-
0.5% NaCl	+	+	-	$+^{W}$	$+^{W}$	$+^{W}$	$+^{W}$	+	+
3% NaCl	+	+	+	+	+	+	+	+	+
8% NaCl	-	-	-	+	+/-	+	+	-	-
10% NaCl	-	-	-	-	-	-	+	-	-
Indole	+	+	+	-	+/-	+	+	+/(-)	+
Arginine	-	-	-	+	+/-	-	-	+/-	+
Ornithine	+	+	$+/+^{D}$	-	-	+	+/-	-	+
Lysine	+	+	+	-	+/-	+	+	-/+	+
Glucose-Gas	-	-	-	-/+	-	-	-	-/+	-
Sucrose	+	-	-	+	+	-	+	+	-
Lactose	$+^{D}/-$	$+^{D}/-$	+	-	+/-	-	-	+/-	+/-
VPR	+/-	-	-	-	+	-	+	+/-	-

+, positive W, weak
-, negative D, delayed
/, or ( ), rare

false-negative oxidase test may be obtained. Therefore, oxidase should be tested either from general purpose media, or with a buffered reagent (27,30), or after centrifugation of a broth subculture (31);

3. Lysine decarboxylase-positive *Aeromonas* strains are being recognized with increasing frequency. While earlier tabulations reported only few (6.5%, 69), several recent studies have found percentages of lysine-positive clinical strains ranging from 73 (34) to 76 (12) to 92.5% (7). In one series, environmental isolates were less frequently lysine-positive than clinical isolates, and *A. hydrophila* less frequently than *A. sobria* strains (13);
4. In the author's experience, deoxyribonuclease activity may be delayed in some strains beyond 24 hours; and
5. Very recently, inositol-positive strains of *A. hydrophila* have been isolated from river water (59).

A new medium for the rapid presumptive identification of *A. hydrophila* was devised by Kaper et al. (35). Mannitol and inositol fermentation, ornithine decarboxylation and deamination, indole production, motility, and H_2S production can be detected in one tube and serve to separate *Aeromonas* from *Klebsiella, Proteus* and other enteric species. The fastest test to differentiate *Aeromonas* and *Plesiomonas* from *Escherichia coli*, however, remains the oxidase test. Hemolysis on blood agar depends on the species of blood used and occurs in *Aeromonas* as well as in *E. coli* (69) but not in *Plesiomonas*.

II. COLLECTION, CULTURE AND ISOLATION

Optimal transport media for *Aeromonas* and *Plesiomonas* have not been investigated but there is no evidence that stool transport media such as buffered glycerol-saline or Cary-Blair medium are insufficient.

A problem arises when the organisms have to be selected from mixed cultures, e.g., stool. A recent study from this laboratory (70) has tested several media developed over the past 15 years for use with human stools (Table 2). The most recent media, MacConkey Agar with trehalose (instead of lactose) (34) and MacConkey Agar with Tween 80 (29) were not included.

Although growth of 23 strains of *Aeromonas* and 10 strains of *Plesiomonas* was excellent on MacConkey Agar, this medium could not be used for differential purposes because both genera contain lactose-positive and lactose-negative strains (69). PBG (42) was found impractical because of the use of agar overlay, poor inhibition of normal stool flora, and poor separation of coliforms from *Aeromonas* and *Plesiomonas*. On SSXLD (49), starch hydrolysis by *Aeromonas* could not be recognized in mixed flora. Media containing ampicillin (DNTA (73), PXA (48), RC (47), TSBA) were unsuitable for *Plesiomonas* because of the occasional sensitivity of this organism to ampicillin (see below). Even DNTA caused a reduction of CFUs by > 1 log in 11 of the *Aeromonas* strains. In artificially contaminated stools, RC showed poor specificity for *Aeromonas*. RS (61) showed the disadvantages of DNTA and RC; in addition, it does not detect lysine-positive strains (34) and does not differentiate between *V. fluvialis* and *Aeromonas* (15). Also, both RC and RS (and presumably DNTA) are unable to differentiate between halophilic strains with GC ratios of 40-49 moles % and *Aeromonas* (16). DFS (55) showed poor sensitivity for *Plesiomonas* and loss of predictive value at high coliform counts. The most sensitive and specific media were: IBG (58), DFS (55), XDC (62) and PXA (48) for *Aeromonas* and IBG and XDC for *Plesiomonas*. APW proved optimal as enrichment broth. In all instances, 0.001 ml of a stool dilution of 1:10 had been plated in order to arrive at separate colonies. Direct oxidase testing by transfer of colonies from plates to a reagent-soaked filter paper was possibly only for IBG, PXA, and XDC, for the reasons mentioned in I.

Table 2. Selective/Differential Media for Aeromonas/Plesiomonas

Medium	Abbrev	Reference	Inhibitor	Differential	Purpose	Tried[c]
Dextrin-fuchsin-sulfite agar	DFS	Schubert, 1967	Na. sulfite, Fuchsin	Dextrin	Water-A[a]	+
DNase test agar + toluidine blue + ampicillin	DNTA	von Graevenitz & Zinterhofer, 1970	Ampicillin	DNAse	Stool-A	+
Inositol-brillant green-bile salts-agar	IBG	Schubert, 1977	Brilliant green, bile salts	Inositol	Stool-P[b]	-
Peptone-beef extract-glycogen agar	PBG	McCoy & Pilcher, 1974	Na. lauryl sulfate	Glycogen	Multi-purpose A	-
Pril-xylose-ampicillin agar	PXA	Rogol et al., 1978	Pril, ampicillin	Xylose	Stool-A	+
Rimler-Shotts agar	RS	Shotts & Rimler, 1973	Citrate, novobiocin, desoxycholate	Lysine, ornithine, maltose	Multi-purpose-A	-
Rippey-Cabelli agar	RC	Rippey & Cabelli, 1979	Ampicillin, desoxycholate, ethanol	Trehalose	Water-A	+
Salt-starch-xylose-lysine-desoxycholate agar	SSXLD	Roland, 1978	Desoxycholate, citrate, NaCl 1.5%	Lysine, starch, xylose	Stool-vibrio	-
Xylose-desoxycholate-citrate agar	XDC	Shread et al., 1980	Citrate, desoxycholate	xylose	Stool-A	-
Alkaline peptone water	APW	Shread et al., 1980	pH 8,5	-	Stool-Vibrio	+
Trypticase soy broth + ampicillin	TSBA	von Graevenitz & Bucher, 1981	Ampicillin	-	Stool-A	+

[a]A, Aeromonas. [b]P, Plesiomonas. [c]By reference source.

III. SEROLOGY

Serological investigations of *Aeromonas* were briefly reviewed in an earlier summary (69). Recent studies (22,37) revealed not only a considerable heterogeneity but also large percentages of strains (61-72%) that could not be grouped with the particular antisera produced. In one epidemic investigation of *Plesiomonas*, 106 (35%) of 302 strains could not be serotyped (3). The authors found 50 serovars (30 O and 11 H antigens) in water sources as well as in stools from diarrhoic patients.

IV. ENTEROTOXIC PROPERTIES

A variety of toxic substances has been isolated from *Aeromonas* strains. At present, there is some difficulty in evaluating reports of various groups working in the field, due to:

1. Lack of standardization of tests for enterotoxigenicity, particularly the rabbit intestinal loop and mouse adrenal Y1 cell tests; and
2. possible interference of other toxic substances, particularly hemolysins and cytotoxins, in enterotoxin assays (39).

The most recent characterization of *Aeromonas* enterotoxin was undertaken by Ljungh (39). The enterotoxin is separate from two hemolysins (A and B) and gives positive reactions in the ileal loop test ($\geq$1 ml/cm, maximum after 16 hours), the rabbit skin test and the adrenal Y1 cell test. Its effects in all three test systems can be separated from those of hemolytic and cytotoxic factors by prior heating (56° 10 min.) or by specific antihemolysin (74). The enterotoxin is cytotonic, i.e., it induces steroidogenesis and increases intracellular cAMP in Y1 cells. Thus, it seems to act similar to cholera toxin. Suckling mouse tests were found negative by the authors. Neutralization experiments with antitoxin to the heat-labile toxins of *V. cholerae* and *E. coli* (LT) did not show cross-neutralization of *Aeromonas* enterotoxin. Also, gangliosides did not block enterotoxic activity. The enterotoxin is heat-labile (80° 10') (74). Ljungh's group also found that not all *Aeromonas* strains carry this enterotoxin which seems to be chromosomal (12, 39), and that production did not correlate with fermentation of certain carbohydrates or certain enzymatic profiles (40) (lysine decarboxylase, however, was not specifically mentioned). Two strains of *Plesiomonas* were loop-negative and positive only in the Y1 cell test (40).

Sanyal et al. (54) had found 12 of 14 *Aeromonas* strains from environmental and fecal cultures to give positive ileal loop tests (1-2 ml per cm after 18 hrs) when $\geq 10^4$ live cells were injected, while six *Plesiomonas* strains were loop-negative. Annapurna and Sanyal (2) found this non-dialyzable "enterotoxic factor" also in cell-free culture supernatants, observed its inactivation after heating to 60° for 20 minutes (or 65° for 10 min.), precipitated it with ammonium sulfate, and saw no significant histopathological change in the loops. Dubey and Danyal (18) observed induration and increased capillary permeability in the skin of adult rabbits after application of crude *Aeromonas* filtrates or partially purified enterotoxin which were also inactivated by 60° (30 min.) treatment and neutralized by specific antiserum. Loop activity was at a maximum at pH 8-10 and was abolished at pH 3 in culture filtrates and at pH 4 in crude preparation. The ED_{50} was contained in 25 µg of protein.

Sanyal et al., later on (53) did observe positive ileal loop tests in 13 *Plesiomonas* strains, some requiring prior passages. Fluid accumulation showed a marked increase up to four hours and only a slight increase at 18 hours. Heating to 121° for 10 min. did not affect the outcome of the test. The suckling mouse test was positive for all strains; CHO and Y1 cells were dislodged. The authors conclude that *Plesiomonas* is not invasive (the Serenyi test being negative) and forms at least a heat-stable enterotoxin.

Gurwith and Williams (26), however, found 2 fecal *Plesiomonas* strains negative in the suckling mouse assay while causing 45-60% rounding of Y1, but no cytotoxicity, in HeLa cells.

Donta and Haddow (17) did find cytotoxic, but not enterotoxic activity in *Aeromonas* strains (some of them obtained from Ljungh's group). In particular, steroidogenesis was not found. The intestinal loop effect did not reach 2 ml per cm and was considered negative. The suckling mouse test (> 0.085) was found positive by Janossy and Tarjan (33) in supernatants of 69 to 87 strains of *A. hydrophila*, 9 of 76 *A. punctata ssp. caviae*, and in 5 of 6 *ssp. punctata*. Burke et al. (6) found 80 of 103 *A. hydrophila* supernatants positive in the same assay when the ratio of intestinal weight to remaining body weight *and* production of diarrhea were scored. In a further investigation (7), these authors found a correlation between biotype and enterotoxin production insofar as most of the suckling mouse test positive strains were Voges-Proskauer (VP) positive and arabinose negative. VP positive, arabinose positive strains were mostly non-enterotoxigenic; so was the ssp. *caviae*. 97% of the strains could be correctly classified as enterotoxigenic if a tube hemolysin assay was used as well. The speciation into *A. hydrophila* and *A. sobria* yielded no useful separation with regard to enterotoxigenicity. The investigations of Seidler et al. (60), Boulanger et al. (5), Cumberbatch et al. (12) and Johnson and Lior (33a) were concerned with cytotoxic, hemolytic and enterotoxic activity of *A. hydrophila* and *A. sobria* strains. Two groups did not find cytotonicity in any strain as measured by rounding of Y1 cells. One found cytotoxicity correlated with diarrheal disease (12), the other saw residual cytotoxicity after 56° (10 min.) heating of supernatants (33a) which could be misinterpreted as a cytotonic effect in Y1 cells (*P. shigelloides* formed neither cytotoxin nor enterotoxin). Various numbers of strains, however, were found by the two former groups to be positive in loop, Y1, and suckling mouse assays (5,60). Finally, Daily et al. (13) distinguished between two groups of environmental and clinical strains of *A. hydrophila* and *A. sobria*. Group I strains showed mouse MLDs of $< 10^7$ (i.p.) CFU and cytotoxic (Y1) properties, were lysine or VP-positive or both, piliated, and adhered to human buccal cells. Group II strains did not show the latter characteristics and had MLDs of $\geq 10^7$ CFUs. Enterotoxigenicity (loop activity) was seen in some strains of both groups. Hemolysis on blood agar occurred mostly in group I strains but was not correlated with any species of *Aeromonas*. Clinical strains were more frequently *A. sobria* (fecal strains exclusively so), and environmental strains were more frequently *A. hydrophila*. Correlation between mouse pathogenicity and hemolysin production had been observed earlier by Caselitz and Krebs (8); and piliation by Ljungh (39). The latter author also found negative Serenyi tests in *A. hydrophila* and inability of the strains to induce diarrhea after intragastric administration in rabbits and rats (39). In jejunal perfusion experiments on rats, preincubation with anticholera toxin reduced intestinal secretion induced by *A. hydrophila* broth supernatants, while immunization with cholera toxin protected against fluid secretion caused by *A. hydrophila* (31a).

It is difficult to explain the contradictions between the findings of several groups but it seems likely that the new standards for the detection of enterotoxin proposed by Maneval et al. (40a), if applied to earlier studies, will clarify the question whether there are *Aeromonas* and/or *Plesiomonas* enterotoxins.

V. DIARRHEAL DISEASE DUE TO AEROMONAS AND PLESIOMONAS AND THE CARRIER STATE. RELATIONSHIP TO ECOLOGY

Diarrhea associated with *Aeromonas* (1,4,10,15,19a,23,25,26,28,36, 43,44,50,51,63,64,65,72,75,78) is ubiquitous, affects any age group, occurs in both sexes, and has a peak during summer and fall. The incidence of *Aeromonas spp.* in diarrhoic disease seems to vary. During an epidemic of diarrhea near Vellore, India, 5% of the stools yielded *A. hydrophila* and 6.5% yielded *Plesiomonas* (4). Among 276 children with diarrhea screened in Winnipeg, Canada, one yielded *A. hydrophila* and two, *Plesiomonas* (26). Of 4500 stool cultures from diarrhoic patients examined in Copenhagen, eight yielded *A. hydrophila* (36). In Zurich, we found the organism in four of 254 stool cultures from patients with diarrhea or their contacts (70). In one recently published series, 31% of individuals with travellers' diarrhea in Thailand yielded *A. hydrophila* in their stools (19a), representing the largest contingent of all individuals with enteric pathogens. In most cases, *Aeromonas* represented the predominant organism in the stool flora (it has to be kept in mind that lactose-fermenting *Aeromonas* strains are probably missed by most investigators unless oxidase testing is routinely done (72)). Afebrile as well as febrile cases have been reported. The diarrhea may be non-bloody, bloody, or even choleriform. Vomiting and abdominal pain may or may not be present. Tenesmus has not been observed. The disease seems to be self-limited and lasts from two to five days. Dehydration may occur. To our knowledge, only one case in an infant has been fatal (41). Fecal carriers have been reported: 30 (0.7%) of 4426 children under two years of age in Northern France (9), none in 300 healthy individuals in Germany (55), six in 188 in New England during summer to fall (73).

Plesiomonas diarrhea is more frequent in tropical areas and in Japan, occurs more often in epidemics, and seems to be choleriform more often (1,3,10,11,14,15,24,26,32,38,43,66,68,79). Other symptoms resemble those of *Aeromonas* diarrhea. Carriers have been reported (1,3,21,43,76,77) but are rarer than *Aeromonas* carriers (e.g., 3 of 38454 healthy Tokyo inhabitants (3)).

The ecology of *Aeromonas* and *Plesiomonas* has been reviewed elsewhere (34,55,59,60,69). Both organisms are aquatic in origin and have been recovered from many water sources including sewage and mud. Neither is considered a marine bacterium (34,46). In contrast to *A. hydrophila, Plesiomonas* cannot multiply at temperatures below 8°C (59). Amphibians, reptiles, and fish are living reservoirs for *Aeromonas*. *Plesiomonas* occurs in these animals (particularly river fish) as well (59,67) but also in domestic animals (3,69). Transmission is rare from animal to man; diseases are most frequently water-borne.

VI. ANTIMICROBIAL SUSCEPTIBILITY AND THERAPY

The former review of antimicrobial susceptibilities by the author (69) requires changes and amplifications. In the meantime, ampicillin-sensitive strains of *Aeromonas* have become known but they are in a minority: one of 113 (47) and seven of 190 (60) environmental strains and eight (13) strains when tested with the Kirby-Bauer technique. These strains are also carbenicillin-sensitive. Thirteen of 16 ampicillin-resistant strains in the above series (13) showed beta-lactamase activity. Of 20 strains examined by Fass and Barnishan (20), most were sensitive to piperacillin, mezlocillin, azlocillin, and cefoxitin. Thus far, all strains have been reported sensitive to cefamandole, mecillinam, cefuroxime, moxalactam, gentamicin, tobramycin, sisomycin, netilmicin, amikacin, nitrofurantoin, and sulfamethoxazole-trimethoprim (13,20,69,72). Occasional strains are sensitive to ampicillin and carbenicillin (see above) and resistant to tetracycline, chloramphenicol, colistin, nalidixic acid, kanamycin and streptomycin (13,20,60,72). A majority is resistant to cephalothin and erythromycin (20,60,72). All are resistant to clindamycin and vancomycin (20). Of 45 strains, we (71) found all sensitive to N-formimidoyl-thienamycin (range 0.1-4.0 mcg/ml) and to ceftazidime (0.1-16 mcg/ml), and most susceptible to cefotiam (MIC 90 = 16 mcg/ml), ceftriaxone (MIC 90 = 2 mcg/ml), and cefotaxime (MIC 90 = 0.5 mcg/ml).

Plesiomonas shigelloides seems to be more sensitive to antimicrobials than *Aeromonas*. With the exception of ampicillin and carbenicillin, most of the above drugs are effective (11,46,69,71). In our series, some strains were cefotiam-resistant. The percentage of ampicillin-sensitive strains varies with publications; in large series, 45-55% were sensitive (11,46).

There are no controlled studies of antimicrobial use in diarrhoic disease due to *Aeromonas*, although some patients have received tetracycline. Hydration of the patient, however, seems to have been more important. No data on antimicrobial therapy of *Plesiomonas* diarrhea exist.

REFERENCES

1. E. Aldova, J. Rakovsky, and A. Chovancova, *J. Hyg. Epidemiol. Microbiol. Immunol. (Prague)*, *10*:470 (1966).
2. E. Annapurna and S. C. Sanyal, *J. Med. Microbiol.*, *10*:317 (1977).
3. T. Arai, N. Ikejima, T. Itoh, S. Sakai, T. Shimada, and R. Sakazaki, *J. Hyg.*, *84*:203 (1980).
4. P. Bhat, S. Shanthakumari, and D. Rajan, *Indian J. Med. Res.*, *62*:1051 (1974).
5. Y. Boulanger, R. Lallier, and G. Cousineau, *Can. J. Microbiol.*, *23*:1161 (1977).
6. V. Burke, J. Robinson, R. J. Berry, and M. Gracey, *J. Med. Microbiol.*, *14*:401 (1981).
7. V. Burke, J. Robinsin, H. M. Atkinson, and M. Gracey, *J. Clin. Microbiol.*, *15*:48 (1982).
8. F.-H. Caselitz and D. Krebs, *Zentralbl. Bakteriol. Parasitenk. Infektionskr. Hyg. Abt. I Orig.*, *187*:56 (1962).
9. M. Catsaras and R. Buttiaux, *Ann. Inst. Pasteur Lille*, *16*:85 (1965).
10. B. D. Chatterjee and K. N. Neogy, *Indian J. Med. Res.*, *60*:520 (1972).
11. R. G. Cooper and G. W. Brown, *J. Clin. Pathol.*, *21*:715 (1968).

12. N. Cumberbatch, M. J. Gurwith, C. Langston, R. B. Sack, and J. L. Brunton, *Infect. Immun., 23:*829 (1979).

13. O. P. Daily, S. W. Joseph, J. C. Coolbaugh, R. I. Walker, B. R. Merrell, D. M. Rollins, R. J. Seidler, R. R. Colwell, and C. R. Lissner, *J. Clin. Microbiol., 13:*769 (1981).

14. W. A. Davis II, J. H. Chretien, V. F. Garagusi, and M. A. Goldstein, *South. Med. J., 71:*474 (1978).

15. W. A. Davis II, J. G. Kane, and V. F. Garagusi, *Medicine, 57:*267 (1978).

16. J. W. Davis and R. K. Sizemore, *Appl. Environ. Microbiol., 42:*544 (1981).

17. S. T. Donta and A. D. Haddow, *Infect. Immun., 21:*(1978).

18. R. S. Dubey and S. C. Sanyal, *Zbl. Bakt. Hyg., I. Abt. Orig. A, 242:*487 (1978).

19. R. S. Dubey and S. C. Sanyal, *J. Med. Microbiol., 12:*347 (1979).

19a. P. Echeverria, N. R. Blacklow, L. B. Sanford, and G. G. Cukor, *J. Infect. Dis., 143:*767 (1981).

20. R. J. Fass and J. Barnishan, *Antimicrob. Agents Chemother., 19:*357 (1981).

21. W. W. Ferguson and N. D. Henderson, *J. Bacteriol. 54:*179 (1947).

22. C. B. Fliermans and T. C. Hazen, *Can. J. Microbiol., 26:*161 (1980).

23. D. Fritsche, R. Dahn, and G. Hoffman, *Zbl. Bakt. Hyg., I. Abt. Orig. A, 233:*232 (1975).

24. E. Geizer, K. Kopecky, and E. Aldova, *J. Hyg. Epidemiol. Microbiol. Immunol., 10:*190 (1966).

25. M. Gurwith, C. Bourque, E. Cameron, G. Forrest, and M. Green, *Arch. Intern. Med., 137:*1461 (1977).

26. M. J. Gurwith and T. W. Williams, *J. Infect. Dis., 136:*239 (1977).

27. A. H. Havelaar, J. C. Hoogendorp, A. J. Wesdorp, and W. A. Scheffers, *J. Microbiol. Serol., 46:*301 (1980).

28. E. B. Helm and W. Stille, *Dtsch. Med. Wochenschr., 95:*18 (1970).

28a. F. W. Hickman, J. J. Farmer III, D. G. Hollis, G. R. Fanning, A. G. Steigerwalt, R. E. Weaver, and D. J. Brenner, *J. Clin. Microbiol., 15:*395 (1982).

29. D. Hoban, W. Forsyth, C. Gratton, and T. Williams, *Abstr. Annu. Meet. Am. Soc. Microbiol.,* C4 (1981).

30. L. K. Hunt, T. L. Overman, and R. B. Otero, *J. Clin. Microbiol.*, *13*:1054 (1981).

31. L. K. Hunt, T. L. Overman, and R. B. Otero, *J. Clin. Microbiol.*, *13*:1117 (1981).

31a. Ch. James, M. Dibley, V. Burke, J. Robinson, and M. Gracey, *Clin. Exp. Immunol.*, *47*:34 (1982).

32. G. Jandl and K. Linke, *Zbl. Bakt. Hyg., I. Abt. Orig. A*, *236*: 136 (1976).

33. G. Janossy and V. Tarjan, *Acta Microbiol. Acad. Sci. Hung.*, *27*:63 (1980).

33a. W. M. Johnson and H. Lior, *Can. J. Microbiol.*, *27*:1019 (1981).

34. J. B. Kaper, H. Lockman, R. R. Colwell, and S. W. Joseph, *J. Aqpl. Bacteriol.*, *50*:359 (1981).

35. J. Kaper, R. J. Seidler, H. Lockman, and R. R. Colwell, *Appl. Environ. Microbiol.*, *38*:1023 (1979).

36. H. Lautrop, *Acta Pathol. Microbiol. Scand. Suppl. 144*, *51*:299 (1961).

37. D. Leblanc, K. R. Mittal, G. Olivier, and R. Lallier, *Appl. Environ. Microbiol.*, *42*:56 (1981).

38. P. L. Lim, *J. Clin. Pathol.*, *31*:223 (1978).

39. A. Ljungh and T. Wadström, *Pharmac. Ther.* *15*:339 (1982).

40. A. Ljungh, M. Popoff, and T. Wadström, *J. Clin. Microbiol.*, *6*:96 (1977).

40a. D. R. Maneval, Jr., R. R. Colwell, S. W. Joseph, R. Grays, and S. T. Donta, *J. Tissue Cult. Methods*, *6*:85 (1980).

41. R. Martinez-Silva, M. Guzmann-Urrego, and F.-H. Caselitz, *Z. Tropenmed. Parasitol.*, *12*:445 (1961).

42. R. H. McCoy and K. S. Pilcher, *J. Fish. Res. Board Can.*, *31*: 1553 (1974).

43. V. Pauckova and A. Fukalova, *Zbl. Bakt. I. Abt. Orig.*, *206*:212 (1968).

44. J. A. Phillips, H. E. Bernhardt, and S. G. Rosenthal, *Pediatrics*, *53*:110 (1973).

45. M. Popoff and M. Véron, *J. Gen. Microbiol.*, *94*:11 (1976).

46. C. Richard, M. Lhuillier, and B. Laurent, *Bull. Inst. Pasteur*, *76*:187 (1978).

47. S. R. Rippey and V. J. Cabelli, *Appl. Environ. Microbiol.*, *38*: 108 (1979).

48. M. Rogol, I. Sechter, L. Grinberg, and Ch. B. Gerichter, *J. Med. Microbiol., 12:*229 (1979).

49. F. P. Roland, *Med. Microbiol. Immunol., 163:*241 (1977).

50. R. Rosner, *Am. J. Clin. Pathol., 42:*402 (1964).

51. A. Samb, J.-P., Chiron, F. Denis, A. Sow, E.-H.-I. Diop, and I. Diop Mar, *Nouv. Presse Méd., 6:*2520 (1977).

52. S. C. Sanyal, L. Ljungh, and T. Wadström, *Zbl. Bakt. Hyg., I. Abt. Orig. A, 248:*384 (1980).

53. S. C. Sanyal, B. Saraswathi, and P. Sharma, *J. Med. Microbiol., 13:*401 (1980).

54. S. C. Sanyal, S. J. Singh, and P. C. Sen, *J. Med. Microbiol., 8:*195 (1975).

55. R. H. W. Schubert, *Arch. Hyg., 150:*688 (1967).

56. R. H. W. Schubert, in *Bergey's Manual of Determinative Bacteriology,* 8th ed. (R. E. Buchanan and N. E. Gibbons, eds.), The Williams & Wilkins Co., Baltimore, 1974, p. 345.

57. R. H. W. Schubert, in *Bergey's Manual of Determinative Bacteriology,* 8th ed. (R. E. Bachanan and N. E. Gibbons, eds.), The Williams & Wilkins Co., Baltimore, 1974, p. 348.

58. R. H. W. Schubert, *Ernst Rodenwaldt-Arch., 4:*97 (1977).

59. R. H. W. Schubert, *Zbl. Bakt. Hyg., I. Abt. Orig. B, 172:*528 (1981).

60. R. J. Seidler, D. A. Allen, H. Lockman, R. R. Colwell, S. W. Joseph, and O. P. Daily, *Appl. Environ. Microbiol., 39:*1010 (1980).

61. E. B. Shotts, Jr. and R. Rimler, *Appl. Microbiol., 26:*550 (1973).

62. P. Shread, T. Donovan, and J. Lee, *Soc. Gen. Microbiol. Quart., 8:*184 (1981).

63. G. Simon and A. von Graevenitz, *Publ. Health Laborat., 27:*159 (1969).

64. C. J. Soussy, F. J. Squinazi, and J. Duval, *Med. Mal. Infect., 5:*11 (1975).

65. S. Stephen, K. N. A. Rao, M. S. Kumar, and R. Indrani, *Ann. Intern. Med., 83:*368 (1975).

66. T. Tsukamoto, Y. Kinoshita, T. Shimada, and R. Sakazaki, *J. Hyg., 80:*275 (1978).

67. L. R. van Damme and J. Vandepitte, *Appl. Environ. Microbiol., 39:*475 (1980).

68. J. Vandepitte, A. Makulu, and F. Gatti, *Ann. Soc. belge Méd. trop.*, *54*:503 (1974).

69. A. von Graevenitz, in *Manual of Clinical Microbiology*, 3rd ed. (E. Lennette, A. Balows, W. Hausler, J. Truant, eds.), American Society for Microbiology, Washington, D.C., 1980, p. 220.

70. A. von Graevenitz and C. Bucher, *J. Clin. Microbiol. 17*:16 (1983).

71. A. von Graevenitz and C. Bucher, *Infection 10*:293 (1982).

72. A. von Graevenitz and A. H. Mensch, *New Engl. J. Med.*, *278*:245 (1968).

73. A. von Graevenitz and L. Zinterhofer, *Health Lab. Sci.*, *7*:124 (1970).

74. T. Wadström, A. Ljungh, and B. Wretlind, *Acta Pathol. Microbiol. Scand. Sect. B*, *84*:112 (1976).

75. I. Wassum, *Zbl. Arbeitsmed. Arbeitsschutz*, *17*:313 (1967).

76. F. W. Winton, *J. Pathol. Bacteriol.*, *95*:562 (1968).

77. H.-H. Wuthe, *Zbl. Bakt. Hyg.*, *I. Abt. Orig. A*, *220*:546 (1972).

78. J. Zajc-Satler, *J. Med. Microbiol.*, *5*:263 (1972).

79. J. Zajc-Satler, A. Z. Dragas, and M. Kumelj, *Zbl. Bakt. Hyg.*, *I. Abt. Orig. A*, *219*:514 (1972).

5

Antibiotic-Associated Enterocolitis

ROBERT FEKETY
Division of Infectious Diseases
Department of Internal Medicine
University of Michigan Medical School University Hospital
Ann Arbor, Michigan

I. INTRODUCTION

When patients develop diarrhea while receiving antibiotics, the differential diagnosis includes a benign, self-limited diarrhea of unknown cause, enterocolitis, and coincidental diarrhea of unrelated cause. Almost all of the enterocolitis caused by antibiotic use is due to overgrowth or superinfection of the intestinal tract with toxigenic *Clostridium difficile* (1). This occurs because of the selective pressure of antibiotics that inhibit and alter the normal flora, especially in the colon. When severe, the illness is characterized by formation of a pseudomembrane that adheres to the inflamed mucosa. Many patients, especially those diagnosed early, have only a friable, congested, inflamed mucosa and are diagnosed as having non-specific colitis by the endoscopists (2). In my experience, approximately 85 per cent of antibiotic-associated diarrhea is self-limited and benign, 8 per cent is associated with non-specific colitis, and 7 per cent with pseudomembraneous colitis. More than 99 per cent of the pseudomembranous colitis is associated with *Clostridium difficile*. Rare cases may have been caused by *Staphylococcus aureus*, *Clostridium perfringens* type C, *Listeria monocytogenes*, or other organisms (2). About 50 per cent of the non-specific colitis is caused by *Clostridium difficile*.

II. DIAGNOSIS OF CLOSTRIDIUM DIFFICILE COLITIS

A. Clinical

High fever, severe abdominal pain, localized tenderness, hematochezia, and polymorphonuclear leukocytosis suggest the diagnosis of enterocolitis rather than benign diarrhea. However, many patients with early or mild Clostridial colitis have watery diarrhea, and cannot easily be distinguished clinically from those with benign diarrhea.

B. Radiological

Barium enema X-ray studies, especially when done with air contrast techniques, may reveal thumbprinting, edema and other abnormalities suggestive of *C. difficile* colitis, but these findings are not specific. Furthermore, radiological examinations are positive most often in severe or advanced illness, in which case they may be dangerous and precipitate toxic megacolon, obstruction, bacteremia, or perforation. Radio-gallium scans have been used to identify localized areas of inflammation in the colon, but are of limited value since gallium is normally eliminated from the body via the intestines. Recently, autologous leukocytes labeled with radioactive indium, which is not eliminated via the intestines, has been useful in determining the site and extent of inflammation in the colon. Scans may be especially useful for those patients who have pseudomembranes too high in the colon to be detectable by sigmoidoscopy.

C. Fecal Leukocytes

Approximately 50 per cent of patients with pseudomembranous colitis have abnormal numbers of white blood cells in a single stained smear of diarrheal stools. This simple procedure is a very useful screening test, for a positive result rules out the benign form of diarrhea and indicates the need for further study and possible specific therapy. However, other infections are also associated with fecal leukocytes, and a negative test does not rule out *C. difficile* colitis. It is rare to find large numbers of organisms resembling *C. difficile* in Gram stains of stools from these patients, so looking for them specifically is not particularly helpful. However, the finding of large numbers of Gram-positive cocci suggests the diagnosis of staphylococcal enterocolitis.

D. Culture

Clostridium difficile is usually present in small numbers in stools of healthy carriers. Because it has few visual characteristics that distinguish it on artificial media from other more numerous organisms, it was formerly difficult to isolate, and was named accordingly, even though it is not very fastidious or aero-sensitive. Fortunately, it is now relatively easy to isolate *C. difficile* from stools using a selective anaerobic medium (CCFA) containing cycloserine (500 μg/ml) and cefoxitin (16 μg/ml) that was developed by George and associates (3). This medium is now commercially available. CCFA is very efficient in detecting the organism in stools from patients with antibiotic-associated colitis, who usually have large numbers of the organism in their stools (10^4 CFU/ml or more). Some other organisms, including clostridia and enterococci, are capable of growing on this medium but they are usually easily distinguished from *C. difficile* by experienced persons. Therefore, when CCFA is used, presumptive positive results can often be reported after incubation for 48 hours, and confirmation by biochemical reactions and/or GLC analysis of fatty acid fermentation products can be accomplished in another 48 hours (4). Another useful confirmatory test is performed by picking isolated suspicious colonies and testing them for their ability to produce the cytotoxin characteristic of *C. difficile*. We have recently developed a modification of CCFA that contains taurocholate and appears better in detection of the spore form of the organism (5).

There are several problems associated with interpretation of stool culture results. The first and most important one is that many healthy persons carry the organism in their stools. Carriage rates of 1 to 5% in healthy adults have been documented (6). Even higher rates have been found in hospitalized patients without diarrhea who have received antibiotics, or are debilitated, or reside in parts of the hospital where the organism is abundant (7). Some patients become healthy carriers after treatment for the disease (8). Thus, the isolation of the organism from a patient with diarrhea does not by itself signify that colitis is also present. This problem is especially acute in newborn nurseries, where carriage rates ranging from 10 to 60 per cent or more have been documented in healthy infants during the first few weeks of life (9). Large amounts of the cytotoxin are also present in the stools of many of these infants, who appear peculiarly resistant to the ill effects of the toxin(s) within their intestinal lumen. The reason for their resistance is not known. Furthermore, some isolates of *C. difficile* are non-toxigenic. This is usually rare, but it is common in some hospitals (10). However, in my experience approximately 85 per cent of *adults* with antibiotic-associated diarrhea who harbor this organism in large numbers in their stools have colitis. A positive culture result may be very helpful, therefore, in deciding whether or not to give the patient specific treatment.

Another potential problem with CCFA that has not been satisfactorily evaluated concerns the fact that some isolates of *C. difficile* are inhibited by the concentrations of cycloserine and cefoxitin that are used in CCFA. This factor may result in the failure to detect the organism in stools of some patients with the disease (11).

Recently, Wilson *et al.* have reported that when sodium taurocholate (0.2 per cent) is added to CCFA, its ability to detect small numbers of spores of *C. difficile* in stools of asymptomatic carriers is enhanced significantly (5).

E. Fluorescent Antibody Tests For The Organism

Wilson et al. reported almost complete success in detecting the organism in the stools of patients with *C. difficile* colitis using an indirect fluorescent antibody test (12). Their antiserum was raised against whole cell preparations. False positive reactions were rare in patients with benign antibiotic-associated diarrhea, but common with stools from healthy persons. Absorption with cross-reacting organisms reduced the sensitivity of the test. This test is rapid and simple, but requires further documentation of its reliability in distinguishing colitis from benign diarrhea.

F. Tests For The Cytotoxin

This test is usually done by demonstrating a cytopathic effect of the toxin in tissue cultures. The test is moderately expensive and not available in many smaller hospitals. While fibroblasts are often employed, many other cell lines have been used in monolayer cultures to demonstrate a rounding effect of the toxic on cells (13,14,15). The toxin action has been called actinomorphic or cytotoxic by some, and cytotonic by others who feel the toxin inhibits but does not kill the cells in which a cytopathic effect is demonstrable. The mechanism of the toxin's action is probably by an effect upon the cell membrane and/or microtubules (16-19). Elucidation of the exact mechanism of action of the cytotoxin has been difficult. It now appears the organism produces at least two toxins, which have been difficult to separate, purify, and characterize (20,21). Toxin mixtures cause fluid secretion in isolated intestinal loops of small animals, and increase capillary permeability in the skin of rodents. The cytotoxin has been called toxin B, while the other toxin, which appears to be lethal for small rodents and to cause intestinal fluid secretion, has been designated toxin A. Antitoxin to toxin A has been relatively easy to raise, but neutralizing antibodies to toxin B, the cytotoxin, have been raised in goats and horses only with difficulty.

Since the rounding of cells in cultures appears to be produced by many different agents, some known and some of unknown nature, demonstration of a cytopathic effect using stool extracts or filtrates is a non-specific finding, although some experienced observers believe they can distinguish the morphologic effects of *C. difficile* toxin from those produced by other agents. Most persons believe that this is not reliable, and that prevention (neutralization) of toxic effects by incubation of the test material with antitoxin is necessary to provide specificity.

Serial dilution of the fecal extracts can be made to determine a toxin titer, but the titer does not correlate well with the severity of the clinical illness in individual patients. It has been speculated that the lack of correlation is due to the possibility that the cytotoxin is not itself the cause of symptoms. It may be attributable in part to improper conditions of storage and transport of the specimen, since the toxin is heat and acid labile and may be inactivated by certain proteolytic enzymes. Some additional details and practical aspects of the tissue culture assay for the cytotoxin that is used at the University of Michigan are provided in the Appendix (Silva, J., Rifkin, G., and Fekety, R. Unpublished observations).

In our experience, more than 95 per cent of *adults* with antibiotic-associated diarrhea who have *C. difficile* cytotoxin in their stools have colitis. Some of the rest probably have colitis that is in the proximal colon, and not visualizable with endoscopic methods available. Extracts are usually positive even when diluted 1:100 more, but many patients with lower titers have severe diarrhea. Fewer than two per cent of patients with pseudomembranous colitis have negative test results. Thus, a positive test is very useful in management of patients. Most neonates with positive tests for the toxin do not have enterocolitis or any other treatable disease caused by *C. difficile*. However, pseudomembranous colitis has been documented in a 5-week-old infant. We have encountered infants with cryptitis and chronic diarrhea beginning after antibiotic therapy who have positive tests for *C. difficile* toxin and who responded promptly to institution of therapy with oral vancomycin. Obviously, better ways to diagnose and evaluate infants with positive tests are needed. At present, a therapeutic trial in selected infants appears justifiable.

At present there is no practical and satisfactory clinical test for toxin A that is generally available, but an ELISA test may be available soon. We and others have found detection of small amounts of toxin B using cell cultures is more sensitive than detection of small amounts of toxin A using animal lethality bioassays (21).

In general, organisms that produce toxin B also produce toxin A, and vice-versa. Some isolates are much more toxigenic than others, and some colonies picked from a plated isolate are more toxigenic than others.

G. Detection Of Fecal Toxin By Counterimmunoelectrophoresis

Because many laboratories could not undertake to identify cytotoxin in cell cultures, alternate methods such as counterimmunoelectrophoretic (CIE) tests were developed. Initial reports suggested this rapid, simple and inexpensive test was more sensitive with fecal specimens than were cell culture methods (22,23). Recently attention has been called to problems and deficiencies with the CIE test (24-26). Both false negative and false positive tests may occur. The available antisera are impure and may detect antigens of *C. difficile* other than its toxins; other clostridial species may share some of these antigens. Thus, CIE is not reliable in diagnosing colitis, and most investigators believe it is of dubious value as a screening test for detecting the organism and/or its toxins.

H. Enzyme Immunoassays for Antigens in Feces

Yolken and associates have devised a sensitive double-antibody enzyme immunoassay for the detection of *C. difficile* antigen in stool specimens (27). Specific *C. difficile* antiserum was used. The method was rapid, simple, highly sensitive, and rarely falsely-positive (less than two per cent). Cross-reactions with *C. sordellii*, *C. bifermentans* and *C. sporogenes* antigens may occur. Further confirmation of the clinical utility of this test is still needed.

I. Gas-Liquid Chromatography

C. difficile isolates produce various fatty acid metabolites, as do other Clostridia. GLC was used to detect one of these, isocaproic acid, in stools from patients and controls. Sensitivity in identifying *C. difficile* positive stools was only 61 per cent, but specificity was good. At best, this procedure might be used as a screening test, but methodological improvements might make it more useful (28).

J. Endoscopy

Proctosigmoidoscopy is the most rapid and reliable way to diagnose pseudomembraneous colitis. Direct visualization of the characteristic lesions, with or without confirmatory biopsy, justifies immediate specific treatment in seriously ill patients. However, this procedure also has problems associated with its discomfort, potential danger, cost, availability and reliability when performed by someone unfamiliar with the lesions. In addition, many patients with diarrhea present only with the findings of non-specific coli tis, and in them biopsy, cultures, toxin tests, and observation of response to therapy may be needed for establishment of a diagnosis. Patients with mucosal hyperemia, friability, and inflammation should have a biopsy performed if possible. Prompt, specific treatment of patients with nonspecific colitis is justified if they have antibiotic-associated diarrhea and are seriously ill. Estimates are that three per cent or more of patients with pseudomembranous colitis have colonic lesions not detectable by sigmoidoscopy because they are above the reach of the sigmoidoscope. Colonoscopy is being performed more and more routinely in order to diagnose these patients.

K. Immunologic Diagnosis

Demonstration of serum antibody responses to *C. difficile* antigens in convalescence is currently not feasible. While antitoxin has been demonstrated in human sera (29), we were unable to detect antitoxin in convalescent sera from 21 patients with the disease, including patients who experienced recurrences (30).

III. CONCLUSION

A simple and reliable diagnostic test for *C. difficile* colitis is not available. Most patients with antibiotic-associated diarrhea do not require therapy with oral vancomycin, metronidazole, bacitracin, or cholestyramine (8). Discontinuation of the precipitating antibiotics, fluid replacement, and avoidance of antiperistaltic agents will suffice in most patients. Many gastrointestinal conditions can resemble *C. difficile* colitis, and seriously ill patients with high fever and leukocytosis should be studied with the most appropriate diagnostic tests available. A screening test for the presence of fecal leukocytes may be helpful, especially in ruling out benign diarrhea. Stool cultures and tests for fecal toxins may be useful in management, but are not as reliable as endoscopy in establishing a diagnosis of colitis. Newer and more practical diagnostic tests are being developed and evaluated, and may make diagnosis and management easier in the near future.

APPENDIX: UNIVERSITY OF MICHIGAN ASSAY PROCEDURE FOR C. DIFFICLE CYTOTOXIN

A. Collecting and Transporting Stool Specimens

1. At least 5 gm (if solid) or 5 ml (if watery) of stool should be provided. An adequate amount of stool is required to insure sufficient toxin to give positive results;
2. The shorter the time between collection and processing of specimens, the more reliable the results. If additional tests are necessary or if the test cannot be completed within a few hours of collection, the specimen should be frozen (preferably at -70°C). The specimen should be thawed only once before a filtrate is made. *Clostridium difficile* cytotoxin deteriorates with repeated freezing and thawing. It remains stable for as long as a week at -15°C, but is most stable when frozen at -70°C. For shipment, the stool should be encased in dry ice and packed in a styrofoam box.

B. Preparation of Fecal Filtrates

1. Place 5-20 gm or ml of stool in a sterile centrifuge tube using a sterile tongue depressor; add an equal amount of phosphate buffered saline (pH 7.2). Sterile centifuge tubes and tongue blades are utilized to avoid contamination of the specimen by bacteria and toxic substances;
2. The mixture is vortexed and centrifuged at 1,400 × gravity for 30 minutes. A second spinning of the supernate at 27,000 × gravity for 30 minutes is usually required, and is desirable to remove organisms and food particles;
3. The supernatant fluid is passed through a sterile 0.45 micron filter and placed in 2 sterile test tubes. Filtration is done to prevent contamination of the system, thus preventing some "false positive" readings. One tube is kept at 4°C for testing as soon as possible. The other tube is stored at -70°C, or if this is not feasible at -15°C. If repeat testing is required, the 4°C tube can be used for up to 48 hours. For later tests, the frozen filtrate should be thawed.

C. Preparation of Cell Cultures

Tissue cultures are used to examine stool filtrates and other specimens such as filtrates of broth cultures of clostridial isolates.

Preparation of Cell Cultures:

1. Cell cultures are prepared in flat-bottom sterile microtiter plates with a capacity of 0.3 milliliters using stock cultures of Walker rat carcinoma (LLC-WRC 256 [ccl 38]) and human foreskin fibroblasts or any other fibroblast line. The most accurate endpoints are determined in flat-bottom microtiter trays; round bottoms may give confusing results. Tissue culture tubes are also satisfactory, although the amount of media and cells are far greater than with the microtiter system.
   Culture Source: American Type Culture Collection, 12301 Parklawn Drive, Rockford, Maryland 20852;
   Type of tissue culture flask: Stock cells are grown on the flat side of a plastic flask which has a surface area of 75 cm^2 and 250 ml total volume;
   Culture media (should be sterile): Gibco Company #320-1885, 3175 Stanley Road, Grand Island, NY 14072; Delbecco's Modified Eagles' Media;
   Additions: 5% (v/v) Fetal Calf or Bovine Serum, Penicillin 100 units/ml, Gentamicin 48 micrograms/ml.

2. Decent spent media from monolayer stock cultures of cell lines.

   For fibroblast cells, wash cells twice with sterile PBS (10 ml × 2) before trypsinizing. Trypsinize with 4 ml prewarmed (37°C) 0.25% trypsin solution prepared in Hanks Balanced Salt solution (without Ca^{++} and Mg^{++}) with 5×10^{-4}M EDTA added. Let trypsin coat cells for about 30 seconds, then decant 3.0 - 3.5 ml. Incubate flask at 37°C for about 3-5 minutes or until cells visually round-up and lift off the bottom of the flask.

   Walker rat carcinoma cells are harvested by cold shocking for one hour at 4°C after adding 15 ml of fresh, prewarmed media. The cells will lift off from the flask after vigorous shaking.

   Trypsin causes proteolysis of the material that permits cells to adhere to the surface of the tissue culture flask and to one another. Trypsinization gently disrupts this monolayer. Other proteolytic enzymes or physical methods may be used for this purpose;

3. After trypsinization, add 15 ml of Delbecco's Modified Eagle's Media to the flask. This solution contains either 5% commercial fetal calf or bovine serum and also antibiotics. Cells are then aspirated off the flask with fresh media. The proteins contained in fetal calf or bovine serum inactivate trypsin and prevent further proteolysis and injury of the cells which have lifted off the monolayer;

4. (a) 0.1 ml of this cell suspension (usually equals 2×10^6 cells/ml) is dispensed into each of the wells of a flat-bottomed microtiter plate and incubated for 24-48 hours at 37°C in 5% CO_2 and humidified atmosphere. This time period allows for the development of a uniform monolayer of cells.

   (b) 5 ml of the suspended cells are added to 10 ml of Delbecco's Modified Eagles' Media in a new flask and incubated at 37°C when a continual line of cells is desired for future tests. Erratic results are obtained after 25-30 serial passages. Therefore, in order to provide stock lines for subsequent cultures, it is necessary to grow several large flasks of cells at one time, to harvest them and then place cell suspensions in small vials for freezing and storage.

D. Cytotoxicity Assay

1. After a monolayer has developed, the microtiter wells are inoculated with 0.1 ml (100 microliters) of undiluted fecal

filtrates and a 10^{-1} dilution (v/v) in phosphate buffered saline (pH 7.2). If there is not enough filtrate to inoculate both cell lines, use fibroblasts only. If only fibroblasts are used, it is desirable to perform the test in duplicate. The fecal filtrate, which may or may not contain toxin, is exposed to the cellular monolayer in order to cause cytopathic changes which are used to determine the end-point (see below);

2. 100 microliters of undiluted filtrate is also added to approximately 5 U of *Clostridium sordellii* (or *C. difficile*) antitoxin and the mixture is incubated for 20-30 minutes at room temperature. Following incubation, 100 microliters of this filtrate-antitoxin mixture is added to a well containing cultured cells. If prevention of the cytopathic effect (neutralization) occurs, then the cytopathic effect is attributed to *Clostridium difficile* toxin;

3. Equine *Clostridium sordellii* antitoxin is cross-reactive with *C. difficile* toxin and is obtained from Bureau of Biologics, Food and Drug Administration, Bethesda, MD 20014; or from Burroughs Wellcome & Company in England. *C. difficile* antitoxin is equally satisfactory and is obtainable from Tracy Wilkins, Ph.D., Anaerobe Research Laboratory, Virginia Polytechnic Institute, Blacksburg, Virginia;

4. The plates are incubated at 37°C in 5% humidified CO_2 and read at 6 and 24 hours by phase microscopy. However, a standard microscope may be used if viewing is with reduced light. Reading the endpoint at 18 to 24 hours gives the most reliable results, although with some specimens cytopathic effects may be seen after only 4 to 12 hours of incubation;

5. The endpoint for a positive test showing toxicity is when 50% or greater of the monolayer displays typical changes. Typical cytopathic changes consist of cell rounding, stringing of cellular processes and disruption of the monolayer. The specificity for *Clostridium difficile* cytotoxins is established when 50% or greater reduction occurs in the cytopathic effects in the well containing the toxin-antitoxin mixture compared with wells containing toxin. Additional serial dilutions may be done if the filtrate has a high titer of toxin, using the highest dilution of fecal filtrate that gave a positive cytotoxic effect. Since the limiting amount of *Clostridium sordellii* antitoxin is employed, fecal filtrates containing large amounts of cytotoxin may produce a negative neutralization test. Serial dilutions are used to determine the amount of toxin in the filtrate to define the exact endpoint for neutralization tests;

6. A known (standard) *Clostridium difficile* toxin can be used in both tissue culture lines to provide a positive test result and also as a control on efficacy of the *Clostridium sordellii* antitoxin. A known toxin standard insures that the cells in the monolayer are sensitive to the toxin.

*Method developed by J. Silva, G. Rifkin and R. Fekety.

REFERENCES

1. J. Silva and R. Fekety, Clostridial and antimicrobial colitis. *Ann. Rev. Med., 32:*327 (1981).
2. R. Fekety, J. Silva, J. Armstrong, M. Allo, R. Browne, J. Ebright, R. Lusk, G. Rifkin, and R. Toshniwal, Treatment of antibiotic-associated enterocolitis with vancomycin. *Rev. Infect. Dis., 3:*S273 (1981).
3. W. L. George, V. L. Sutter, D. Citron and S. M. Finegold, Selective and differential medium for isolation of *Clostridium difficile. J. Clin. Microbiol., 9:*214 (1979).
4. L. V. Holdeman, E. P. Cato, and W. E. C. Moore, *Anaerobe Laboratory Manual,* 4th Ed. Virginia Polytechnic Institute and State University, Blacksburg, 1977.
5. K. H. Wilson, M. J. Kennedy and F. R. Fekety, Use of sodium taurocholate to enhance spore recovery on a medium selective for *C. difficile. J. Clin. Microbiol., 15:*443 (1982).
6. K. H. Kim, R. Fekety, D. H. Batts, D. Brown, M. Cudmore, J. Silva and D. Waters, Isolation of *Clostridium difficile* from the environment and contacts of patients with antibiotic-associated colitis. *J. Infect. Dis., 143:*42 (1981).
7. R. Fekety, K. H. Kim, D. Brown, D. H. Batts, M. Cudmore and J. Silva, Epidemiology of antibiotic-associated colitis. *Amer. J. Med., 70:*906 (1981).
8. J. Silva, D. H. Batts, R. Fekety, J. F. Plouffe, G. D. Rifkin and I. Baird, Treatment of *C. difficile* colitis and diarrhea with vancomycin. *Amer. J. Med., 71:*815 (1981).
9. D. F. Welch and M. I. Marks, Is *C. difficile* pathogenic in infants? *J. Pediat., 100:*393 (1982).
10. F. R. Fekety and J. Silva, Unpublished observations (1982).
11. R. Fekety, J. Silva, R. Toshniwal, M. Allo, J. Armstrong, R. Browne, J. Ebright and G. Rifkin, Antibiotic-associated colitis: effects of antibiotics upon *Clostridium difficile* and the disease in hamsters. *Rev. Infect. Dis., 1:*386 (1979).

12. K. H. Wilson, J. Silva and R. Fekety, Fluorescent antibody to *C. difficile* as an aid to diagnosis of *C. difficile* colitis. *J. Clin. Microbiol.* (in press).

13. G. D. Rifkin, F. R. Fekety, J. Silva and R. B. Sack, Antibiotic-induced colitis. Implications of a toxin-induced by *C. sordellii* antitoxin. *Lancet, 2:*1103 (1977).

14. T. W. Chang, M. Lauermann and J. G. Bartlett, Cytotoxicity assay in antibiotic-associated colitis. *J. Infect. Dis., 140:*765 (1979).

15. G. D. Rifkin, R. Fekety and J. Silva, Neutralization by *C. sordellii* antitoxin of the toxins implicated in clindamycin-induced cecitis in the hamster. *Gastroenterology, 75:*422 (1978).

16. M. Thelestam and M. Bronnegard, Interaction of cytopathogenic toxin from *C. difficile* with cells in tissue culture. *Scand. J. Infect. Dis., Supple. 22:*16 (1980).

17. S. T. Donta and S. J. Shaffer, Effect of *C. difficile* on tissue cultured cells. *J. Infect. Dis., 141:*218 (1980).

18. S. W. Rothman and J. E. Brown, Inhibition of membrane functions on intact HeLa cells by *C. difficile* cytotoxic culture filtrates. *Curr. Microbiol., 6:*221 (1981).

19. M. J. Gurwith, C. Langston and B. Dunsmore, Morphologic and functional effects of *C. difficile* in tissue culture. *Canad. J. Microbiol., 28:*100 (1982).

20. N. S. Taylor, G. M. Thorne and J. G. Bartlett, Comparison of two toxins produced by *C. difficile*. *Infect. Immun., 34:*1036 (1981).

21. D. M. Lyerly, D. E. Lockwood, S. H. Richardson and T. D. Wilkins, Biological activities of toxins A and B of *C. difficile*. *Infect. Immun., 35:*1147 (1982).

22. D. F. Welch, S. K. Menge and J. M. Matsen, Identification of toxigenic *C. difficile* by counterimmunoelectrophoresis. *J. Clin. Microbiol., 11:*470 (1980).

23. R. W. Ryan, I. Kwasnik, and R. C. Tilton, Rapid detection of *C. difficile* toxin in human feces. *J. Clin. Microbiol., 12:* 776 (1980).

24. R. Poxton and M. D. Byrne, Detection of *C. difficile* toxin by counterimmunoelectrophoresis: a note of caution. *J. Clin. Microbiol., 14:*349 (1981).

25. S. E. H. West and T. D. Wilkins, Problems associated with counterimmunoelectrophoresis assays for detecting *C. difficile* toxin. *J. Clin. Microbiol., 15:*347 (1982).

26. H. G. Levine, M. Kennedy and J. T. LaMont, Counterimmunoelectrophoresis vs. cytotoxicity assay for the detection of *C. difficile* toxin. *J. Infect. Dis., 145:*398 (1982).

27. R. H. Yolken, L. S. Whitcomb, G. Marien, J. D. Bartlett, J. Libby, M. Ehrich and T. Wilkins, Enzyme immunoassay for the detection of *C. difficile* antigen. *J. Infect. Dis., 144:*378 (1981).

28. C. Potvliege, M. Labbe and E. Yourassowsky, Gas-liquid chromatography as screening test for *C. difficile*. *Lancet, 2:*1105 (1981).

29. S. Nakamura, M. Mikawa, S. Nakashio, M. Takabatke, I. Okado, K. Yamakawa, T. Serikawa, S. Okumura and S. Nishida, Isolation of *C. difficile* from the feces and the antibody in the sera of young and elderly adults. *Microbiol. Immunol., 25:*345 (1981).

30. J. Silva, R. Lusk, R. Fekety, K. Wilson, D. Batts, D. Mason and D. Spratt, Immune responses of hamsters and humans with antibiotic-associated colitis. In *Anaerobic Bacteria--Selected Topics*. D. W. Lambe, R. J. Genco, and K. J. Mayberry-Carson (Eds.), Plenum Press. New York. pp. 257, 1980.

6

Laboratory Detection of Enterotoxins

KAYE WACHSMUTH
Molecular Biology Laboratory
Bacterial Disease Division
Center for Infectious Diseases
Centers for Disease Control
Atlanta, Georgia

There are two known primary mechanisms of acute bacterial diarrheas due to infection by gram-negative bacilli. One is an invasion of the intestinal mucosa or epithelial layer, and the other is the production of enterotoxins in the intestinal lumen. Cholera is undoubtedly the prototype of an enterotoxigenic illness during which a patient may lose in excess of 10 liters of fluid per day (13). Although the clinical picture of cholera can range from asymptomatic to severe (cholera gravis), death can result within 24 hours in over half of the untreated cases. *Escherichia coli* and *Vibrio mimicus* can also cause a cholera-like illness in adults and children in many developing countries of the world and in tourists visiting these areas (9,37). Other enteric organisms, such as *Klebsiella, Enterobacter, Aeromonas,* and *Vibrio fluvialis,* produce detectable enterotoxins, but these have not been as clearly implicated in pathogenesis as cholera toxin (CT) and the *E. coli* heat labile (LT) and heat stable (ST) toxins (17,27,28). *Yersinia enterocolitica, Vibrio parahaemolyticus* and at least some shigellae and salmonellae produce toxins but seem to have additional or more complex pathogenic mechanisms (19,22,23,38). Much *Vibrio cholerae* and *E. coli* diarrhea is caused by strains in which neither invasiveness nor toxin production can be demonstrated.

Before discussiong the various toxin assays, it is important to emphasize that the assay results for strains from all of these bacterial species are dependent on the conditions under which the bacteria are cultured. Optimal conditions for toxin production vary from toxin to toxin as well as strain to strain, even within the same genus and species. The El Tor and Classical biotypes of *V. cholerae* serotype 01 have different requirements for optimal toxin elaboration (25). The many non-01 *V. cholerae* isolated from stools or other sites in humans and from the environment are only now being tested in the various pathogenicity assays. For many of these strains there are often very stringent and specific requirements for incubation time, pH, temperature, aeration, carbohydrate substrate, metal ions, and other undefined medium constituents. Optimal growth does not always correspond to peak toxin concentration.

The toxin of *V. cholerae* serotype 01 is one of the most thoroughly investigated enterotoxins and much is known about its structure and physiology at the molecular level (13). In Table 1, some of the basic characteristics of CT are compared with the enterotoxins of *E. coli*. It is apparent that CT and LT are very closely related by all parameters measured. Not included in this table is the fact that plasmid DNA determining the production of LT does hybridize with chromosomal DNA in the toxigenic vibrios. Also, amino acid sequences and subunit characteristics of CT and LT are similar although not identical (31). Figure 1 shows a diagram of the probable mechanisms of LT and CT action. Both toxins act as

Table 1. Enterotoxin Characterizations

Property	ST*	LT*	CT*
Heat sensitive	-	+	+
Trypsin sensitive	-	+	+
Acid sensitive	-	+	+
Molecular weight	1,972	Approx. 91,000	84,000
Gene(s) location	Transposon (plasmid)	Plasmid	Chromosome
Stimulation of adenyl cyclase	-	+	+
Stimulation of guanyl cyclase	+	-	-
Immunogenic	-	+	+
Neutralized by anti-CT	-	+(1/3)	+
by anti-LT	-	+	+(1/100)
by GM_1	-	+	+
Choleragenoid blocks	-	±	+

*ST = stable toxin, active in the infant mouse
LT = labile toxin
CT = cholera toxin

"promiscuous" hormones and can activate adenyl cyclase in most eucaryotic cells, as indicated in this figure. There are several ST molecules which differ in molecular weight, and amino acid sequences. The ST described in this manuscript is that molecule elaborated by strains of *E. coli* isolated from humans, unless otherwise stated (33).

There are three known types of enterotoxigenic *E. coli* (ETEC). They produce: (i) heat-labile enterotoxin only, (ii) heat-stable enterotoxin only and (iii) both toxins concurrently (LT-ST) (37). *E. coli* enterotoxin production has been demonstrated to be a plasmid-mediated phenomenon (18), with separate plasmid species governing ST production alone, LT alone and LT-ST production (18,44,45).

Since these plasmids can be transferred *in vitro* from one *E. coli* strain to another, it is not unexpected that diverse *E. coli*

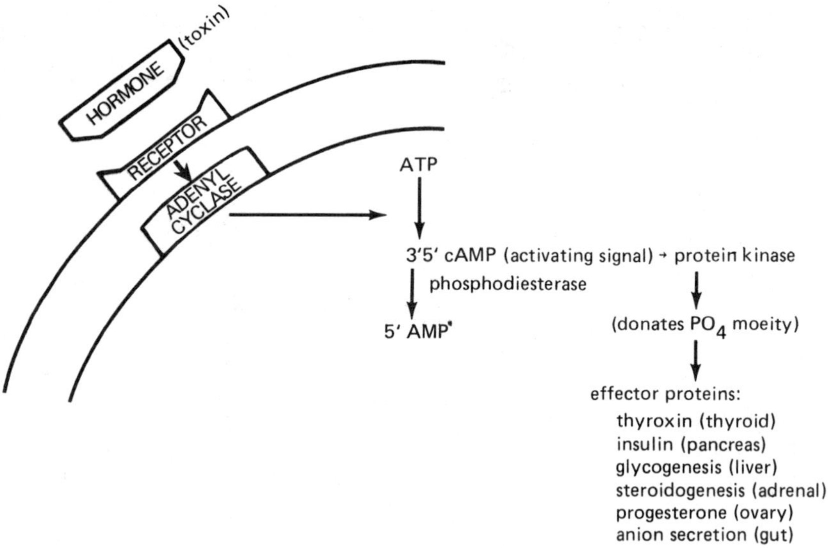

Fig. 1 Activation by cholera and cholera-like toxins of cyclic adenosine monophosphate mediated cell activities. This activation is the basis for intestinal fluid secretion and for the morphological changes used in tissue culture assays (8,16).

serotypes are responsible for diarrheal illness (7,32). Tests to detect enterotoxin production may be as relevant epidemiologically as serotyping and may be more relevant than screening with a very limited number of antisera against the classical enteropathogenic *E. coli* (EPEC) (43). Similarly we have recently found that the 01 serotype of *V. cholerae* is not synonymous with enterotoxigenicity or, thereby, enteropathogenicity (5,21). In cases of apparent *E. coli* or *V. cholerae* infection, the determination of toxin production is an invaluable diagnostic tool. The toxin assays that are known to be available today in research and reference laboratories are described below. The sequence in which they are presented often reflects the evolutionary development of these assays.

The rabbit ileal loop test was the first enterotoxin assay developed; it was initially used for CT but has been adapted for most enterotoxin-producing organisms (3). The assay is performed *in vivo* using ligated segments of rabbit intestine (loops) and is therefore a time-consuming, cumbersome, and expensive test that is not well suited to clinical or most research laboratories, especially where large numbers of *E. coli* strains must be evaluated. In addition, results are difficult to standardize. After exteriorization and ligation of the rabbit small intestine, a cell-free supernate is injected into each ileal loop and the abdomen is closed for 6 or 18 hours. The intestine is then removed, measured, and weighed to determine the amount of fluid accumulation stimulated by the toxin. Results are expressed as volume of fluid per length of intestinal loop. Maximal volume per length ratios occur after 10 hours for LT and CT but after only 4 hours for ST. The assay can be used for toxin neutralization experiments and with whole-cell cultures. All of the loop assays should include both positive and negative controls in each rabbit and two rabbits per culture (with reverse orientation of loop sequences). Many whole-cell cultures give positive loop reactions where filtrates elicit no reaction; these organisms are potentially enteropathogenic but do not necessarily produce an enterotoxin.

The infant rabbit test is also an *in vivo* assay that was originally used for *V. cholerae* (10). It can detect the production of CT, LT, or ST (37). After overnight starvation (5% dextrose is given orally to maintain hydration), 7-day old rabbits are *infected* with the test organism by gastric intubation or by direct intragastric or intralumenal (small intestine) injection. After a 7-hour incubation period, the animals are sacrificed; the intestines are removed and the fluid volume is measured. Results are expressed as a ratio of intestinal fluid in milliliters over remaining intestinal weight in grams. Because it can detect an EPEC toxin isolated from infants with diarrhea when the rabbit ileal loop test is negative (14,26), the infant rabbit test is apparently more sensitive. This model has also been effectively used for the study of colonization potential of human ETEC (11). The main drawbacks are that each culture requires at least three rabbits and that a positive and negative control culture should be included at least once during an investigation. The variability and expense should be considered before this infection model is adopted.

A recently-described assay appears to be a combination of the adult loop and infant rabbit models (41). The assay has been designated the RITARD (removable intestinal tie-adult rabbit diarrhea) model. When the small intestine of an adult rabbit is temporarily ligated so that bacterial cells are not easily cleared, an infection, and fatal diarrhea are produced by *V. cholerae* and ETEC strains. The actual infective processes of these enterotoxigenic organisms may be studied in this system where immune factors in a mature host can also be monitored.

There is another *in vivo* loop method which measures the fluid absorption and/or secretion in the rat intestine. The rat intestinal perfusion assay measures fluid changes by monitoring the concentration of a nonabsorbable marker. This assay has detected enterotoxin production by many species of organisms, including known EPEC. The heat-stable and heat-labile enterotoxins detected here do not seem to be the traditional LT and ST produced by *E. coli*. Many of the positive cultures in this system remain negative in other assays (24).

The rabbit skin test, or vascular permeability factor assay, will detect the presence of either CT or LT, and the activity of both, in this test, can be neutralized by a standardized anticholeragen serum (4). A cell-free culture supernatant of *E. coli* and dilutions of antisera are injected intradermally into the shaved back of a young adult rabbit and are followed 18 hours later by an intravenous injection of Evans blue dye; capillary permeability (bluing) and induration occur if toxin activity is present. The test is sensitive to CT in the range of 0.1-3.5 nanograms per milliliter; however, its precise sensitivity to LT cannot be stated due to the impurity of most LT and specific LT antitoxin preparations that are now available. Although this procedure permits assay of multiple *E. coli* cultures using one rabbit, it remains an *in vivo* test system with attendant disadvantages.

Two tissue culture assays have been developed that can detect CT and LT but not ST. In both assays, a change in cell morphology is known to occur in response to stimulation of adenyl cyclase activity by the toxin. The Chinese hamster ovary (CHO) cell line is sensitive to 10 picograms per milliliter of purified CT (16). The cell-free filtrate of a test culture is mixed with freshly suspended CHO cells and when read after 20-24 hours of incubation can cause elongation of up to 50% of the cell monolayer (16). Test yielding more than 10% elongated cells are considered positive. *Enterobacter, Citrobacter, Salmonella, Klebsiella* and *V. fluvialis* have been reported as positive in the CHO assay (17,28,38).

The other widely used tissue culture method employs the Y-1 clone of mouse adrenal tumor cells and is also sensitive to 10 picograms per milliliter of CT (8). This assay also detects LT in cell-free culture filtrates and can be adapted for use with crude broth cultures when high concentrations of antibiotic are used to prevent bacterial growth. The original procedure measured the amount of steroid produced in response to either CT or LT, and correlated this with a marked cytopathic effect in the Y-1 monolayer which can be used to determine a positive or negative reaction (36). *Aeromonas hydrophila* elicits another, distinctive type of cell rounding which does not seem to require adenyl cyclase activation. Many of the vibrios and other organisms produce extracellular heat-labile products which cause a nonspecific rounding often misinterpreted as being caused by CT (21). It is best to neutralize a positive or doubtful reaction with specific antitoxin or other binding substances such as ganglioside G_{M1}, the known toxin receptor site in host cell membranes. The Y-1 and the CHO assay systems can be used to detect LT and CT neutralizing antibody from the sera of affected patients.

Both methods require some skill, special reagents, and equipment for maintenance of the established cell lines. For both the Y-1 and CHO assays, *E. coli* are grown in trypticase soy broth with 0.6% yeast extract, pH 7.4, (TSBYE) with slight aeration for 24 hours. Culture supernates are filtered through a 0.45 μm membrane before being added to tissue culture monolayers. Vibrios are grown in Craig's medium at 30 C for 24 hours with moderate aeration (25); culture supernates are filtered through a 0.22 μm membrane.

A system as sensitive as tissue culture, but without the limitations of an *in vivo* assay is the enzyme-linked immunosorbent assay (ELISA). The assay relies on many CT reagents because of their purity and availability. Figure 2 diagrams the indirect ELISA method, first described by Yolken (46), used in our laboratories where the microtiter wells are coated with either burro anti-CT or ganglioside G_{M1} (42). Culture supernatants are added to the coated wells. Toxin molecules in the supernatant bind to the previously bound antibody or G_{M1} in the well and react with a second antibody, rabbit anti-CT. Goat anti-rabbit immunoglobulin conjugated to the enzyme alkaline phosphatase is added and reacts with the well-bound second antibody. Finally the enzyme substrate p-nitrophenyl phosphate is added, and the bound enzyme degrades the substrate forming a yellow product which indicates the presence of LT, CT or immunologically related molecules in the culture supernatant. These reactions can be read spectrophotometrically, and a positive or toxigenic culture can be established when the test well has an optical density at least twice that of the negative control wells (46). The primary concern in using this assay exclusively is that a partial or inactive toxin molecule may produce a positive reaction and may not signify toxigenicity or pathogenicity. *E. coli* and other enteric organisms are prepared for ELISA by growth in Evan's CAYE medium, pH 8.5, at 37 C for 48 hours. Vibrios are grown in Craig's medium at 30 C for 24 hours with moderate aeration (25). No filtration of supernates is necessary.

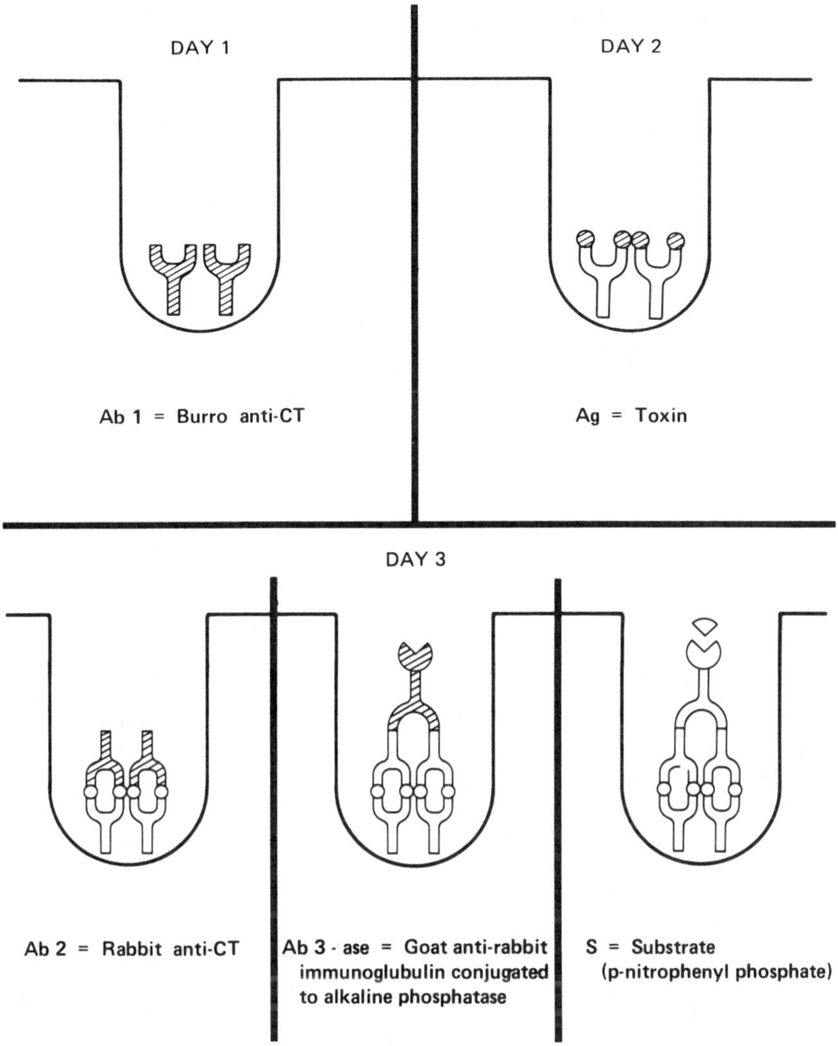

Fig. 2 Schema of an enzyme-linked immunosorbent assay for cholera and cholera-like toxins. If purified *E. coli* labile toxin (LT) is available, LT reagents are more desirable to assay *E. coli* strains. Also, G_{M1} may be substituted for Ab1.

Other immunological assays for CT and LT have been developed within the past 5 years. These include passive immune hemolysis (12), radial immune hemolysis (1), coagglutination with staphylococcal protein A (2) and a radioimmune assay (15). All of these have proven effective in detecting LT and CT and have been adapted by laboratories with varying needs and expertise.

Another assay routinely used in our laboratories is the infant (suckling) mouse assay. It is unique in its ability to detect ST specifically. For human strains of *E. coli* a 24-hour aerated culture supernate, as prepared for tissue culture assays, is mixed with Evans blue dye and injected into the stomach of a 1- to 4-day-old mouse, as shown in Figure 3. After a 3- to 4-hour incubation period at room temperature, the mice are sacrificed, their intestines are removed, and weights are determined. Fluid accumulations are expressed as a ratio of intestinal to remaining body weight (6). The cutoff point between positive and negative ratios is 0.083 (29). Other organisms can produce a positive mouse fluid accumulation but have different growth requirements for toxin elaboration and may act through mechanims other than guanylcyclase (20). *Yersinia entero-*

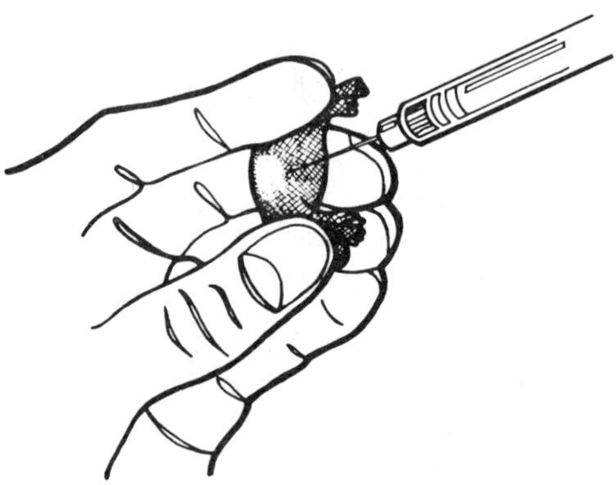

Fig. 3 Intragastic injection of a 3-day-old suckling mouse for the assay of heat-stable toxin. A sterile culture filtrate of the test organism is mixed with Evan's blue dye before injection.

colitica is grown at 25 C in TSBYE for 48 hours and vibrios are grown as described for CT in the ELISA procedure.

One of the newest diagnostic tools is hybridization using genetic probes for enterotoxin. At present there are specific probes for both LT and ST genes (21,30,31). These probes are very small DNA fragments (157-800 base pairs) which contain genes for toxins or toxin subunits. The probe is radiolabeled with ^{32}P and denatured at alkaline pH so that its single-stranded fragment of DNA can associate or hybridize with the toxin genes of test organisms. This is an exquisitely sensitive and specific assay which can actually detect the toxin gene sequences in unpurified cultures grown overnight from a loopful of diarrheal stool (30). When DNA from the test organism is isolated and purified before probing, it is possible to identify the specific plasmid or portion of the chromosome carrying the toxin genes (31,45). The application used most frequently in our laboratory is colony hybridization, which assays the whole cell DNA from growth of a pure culture rather than stool or purified DNA. The old problems of toxin expression and elaboration or possible inactivation are avoided by assaying for the responsible genes. The new problems encountered with any of the present genetic probe methodologies are the hazard of exposure to radioactive isotopes and the rapid decay of radioactivity in the labeled probe.

Current probe techniques are based on the observation that denatured or single stranded DNA binds to nitrocellulose membranes and is "fixed" by baking at 80°C. Stool and colony cultures from diarrheal patients are grown overnight after inoculation directly onto the membrane overlaying an agar medium. The bacterial cells are lysed on the membrane and the resulting DNA is denatured *in situ* when membrane filters, with growth, are placed in an alkaline solution. The DNA (from stool, pure culture or purified preparations) is baked onto the membrane. The filters are subsequently incubated with denatured, labeled probe which hybridizes with its complementary nucleic acid sequence on the solid phase (membrane). After extensive washing to remove excess label and probe, the air dried membranes are exposed to X-ray film overnight at -70°C. The resultant autoradiograph identifies the toxin genes as darkened areas on the exposed X-ray film. Figure 4 is an autoradiograph from the colony hybridization technique used to probe 25 strains of *E. coli* inoculated onto each nitrocellulose membrane.

Under conditions where purified DNA is probed, the DNA from a test organism is electrophoresed through an agarose gel. The DNA is denatured in the gel at alkaline pH and is then chromatographed to a nitrocellulose membrane so that each DNA band within the gel is transferred to the membrane (40). Membranes are treated as described above, and autoradiographs indicate the presence of toxin genes in individual plasmids or chromosome fragments of DNA. Figure 5 is a photograph of plasmid DNA electrophoresed through an agarose gel and the corresponding autoradiograph produced from a Southern blot of that gel (40).

Table 2 summarizes the results of the assays mentioned above for CT, LT, and ST. Table 3 indicates the sensitivity of some of these assays in terms of the quantity of purified CT detectable. One misleading feature in Table 3 is the relatively low sensitivity of the infant rabbit assay; the advantage of this model is that it measures infectivity and may therefore be a more precise reflection of pathogenicity than enterotoxin detection alone.

Although many of these assays are becoming routine in research and reference laboratories, the value of enterotoxin testing in the clinical laboratory is doubtful for several reasons: (a) Although we have seen two well-documented outbreaks of ETEC in the United States (34,35), at CDC we have seen few enterotoxigenic organisms isolated from sporadic episodes of diarrhea (6,7,29). (b) Specific serotypes of *E. coli* (including the two epidemics of ETEC mentioned above), *Y. enterocolitica* and possibly of *V. cholerae* correlate well with pathogenicity. Serotyping with precise reagents would be much more applicable in the clinical setting and may be indicative of more complete pathogenic mechanisms or traits than toxin elaboration alone; e.g., presence of colonizing antigens. Using *E. coli*

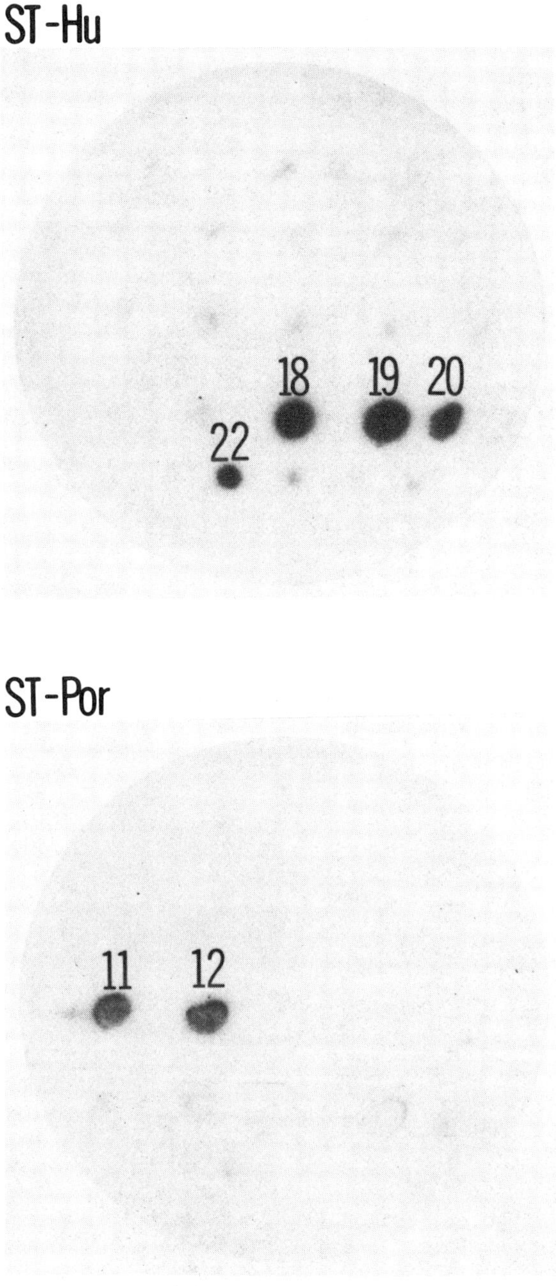

Fig. 4 Colony hybridization (autoradiograph) of twenty-five strains of *E. coli*, in duplicate, with the heat-stable toxin (ST) gene probes derived from human and porcine strains of enterotoxigenic *E. coli*. Colonies numbered 18, 19, 20, and 22 contain the human ST gene sequence, and colonies 11 and 12 contain the porcine ST sequence.

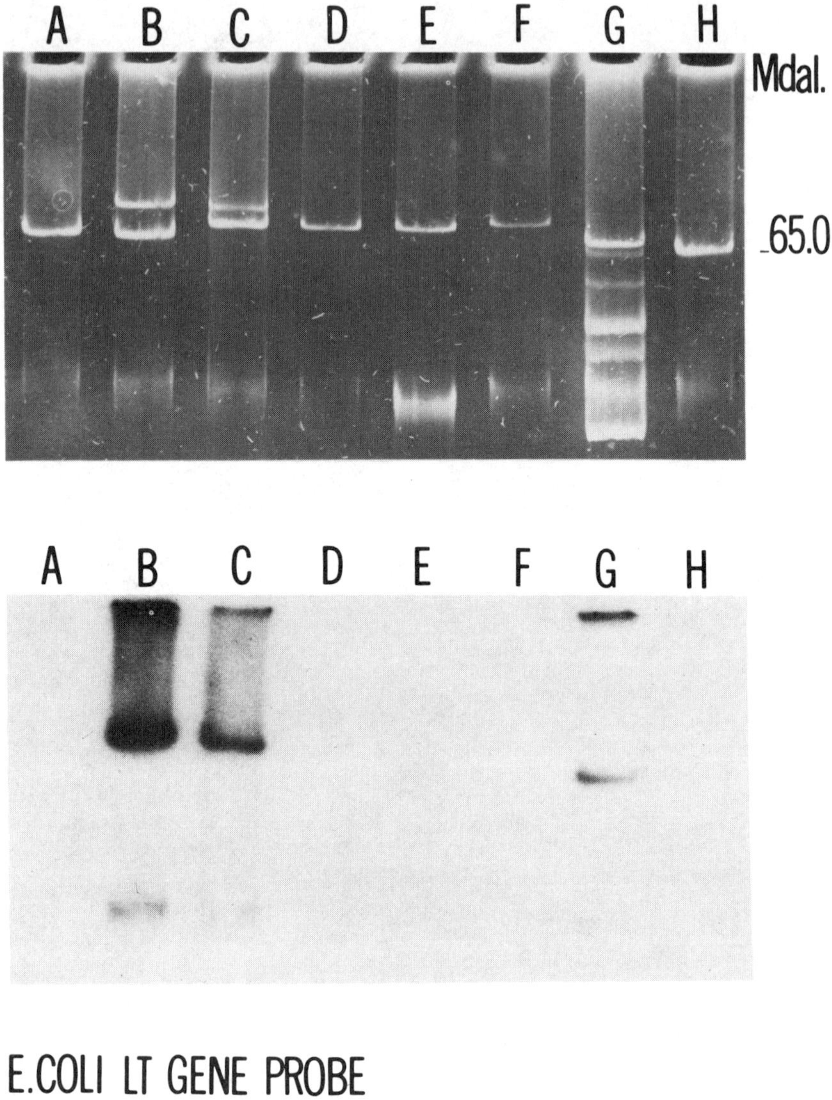

Fig. 5 Agarose gel electrophoresis of plasmid DNA and the corresponding autoradiograph demonstrating the presence of heat-labile toxin gene sequences in the plasmid bands of tracks B, C, and G.

Table 2. Enterotoxin Assays

Assay		ST*	LT*	CT*
Rabbit ileal loop:	6H	+	+	+
	18H	-	+	+
Infant rabbit		+	+	+
Rabbit skin		-	+	+
Infant mouse		+	-	-
Tissue culture†:	CHO	-	+	+
	Y-1	-	+	+
Passive immune hemolysis		-	+	+
Enzyme-linked immunoassay		-	+	+
Radioimmune assay		-	+	+
Genetic probe		+	+	+

*ST = stable toxin
LT = labile toxin
CT = cholera toxin

†CHO = Chinese hamster ovary
Y-1 = Mouse adrenal tumor

Table 3. Sensitivity of Various Assays Used to Measure Cholera Toxin

Assay	Amount of Toxin Eliciting a Positive Response (per ml)
Rabbit ileal loop	30 ng*
Infant rabbit	250-500 ng
Rabbit skin test	0.1-3.5 ng
Chinese hamster ovary tissue	10 pg*
Y-1 mouse adrenal cell tissue culture assay	10 pg
Radioimmune assay	10 pg
Enzyme-linked immunosorbent assay	10 pg

*ng = nanogram
pg = picogram

as an example, Table 4 illustrates the limited number of serotypes associated with toxin production. Table 5 shows that this association is maintained over long periods of time and over diverse geographical locations. This is surprising because toxin genes are known to be located on plasmid DNA. Furthermore, the genes for ST production have been shown to exist on transposable elements (able to insert or delete into non-homologous DNA) located on plasmids (39). On the other hand, there are circumstances, especially with *V. cholerae*, where the determination of toxin production is essential to an evaluation of potential public health hazards. Table 6

Table 4. Serotypes of Enterotoxigenic (ETEC), Enteropathogenic (EPEC), and Enteroinvasive (EIEC) *Escherichia coli**

ETEC		EPEC			EIEC†
06:H16	078:H11	026:H-	086:H-	018:H-	028
06:H-	078:H12	026:H11	086:H34	018:H7	0112
08:H9	0109:H21	055:H-	0119:H6	018:H14	0124
08:H?	0115:H21	055:H6	0124:H-	010:H-	0136
015:H11	0115:H40	055:H7	0124:H30	020:H26	0143
015:H-	0128:H7	0111:H-	0125:H21	020:H34	0144
020:H-	0128:H12	0111:H2	0126:H-	028:H-	0152
025:H42	0128:H21	0111:H12	0126:H9	044:H18	0164
025:H-	0148:H28	0111:H21	0128:H2	044:H34	
027:H20	0149:H19	0127:H-	0128:H7	0112:H-	
063:H-	0159:H4	0127:H9	0128:H12		
063:H12	0159:H20	0127:H21			

*Adapted from reference 43.

†Although EIEC are often non-motile, most references do not include H antigen serotyping. In general, these strains can cause an illness indistinguishable from bacillary dysentery and share common antigens with *Shigella*.

Table 5. Isolation of *Escherichia coli* 06:H16

Location	Year	Source	LT	ST	R
Aden	1966	AD[1]	+	+	Su
Sharjan	1969	AD	+	+	-
United Kingdom	1969	ID[2]	+	+	
United Kingdom	1970	ID	-	-	Su
Ethiopia	1972	AD	+	+	-
Worcester	1973	OAD[3]	+	+	-
Hong Kong	1975	AD	+	+	SM
	1975	AD	+	-	-
Canada	1975	ID	+	+	-
Gloucester	1976	OID[4]	+	+	-
Canada	1976	ID	+	+	-
Oregon	1976	OAD	+	+	-
Wisconsin	1980	OAD	+	+	TC

[1] Adult diarrhea
[2] Infant diarrhea
[3] Outbreak of adult diarrhea
[4] Outbreak of infant diarrhea

shows that serotype alone does not constitute perfectly or predict accurately production of CT, yet *V. cholerae* 01 strains have been the only strains associated with pandemic cholera. In the case of 01 isolation by hospital or state laboratories, cultures should be sent to a reference laboratory.

(c) Although such organisms as *Shigella, Salmonella, V. parahaemolyticus* and *Y. enterocolitica* do produce an enterotoxin, there appears to be little correlation between this and the clinical syndrome. Mechanisms of penetration and invasion may be more important in their pathogenesis. (d) The simplified and refined *in vitro* assays, such as ELISA, radioimmune assay, or passive immune hemolysis, which measure specific toxins and are most adaptable to

Table 6. Pathogenesis of *Vibrio* Species Associated with Human Disease

1. *Vibrio cholerae*, serotype 01	(a) produces cholera toxin (b) nontoxigenic
2. *Vibrio cholerae*, non-01	(a) produces toxin similar to cholera toxin (b) produces a heat-stable toxin (c) invasive (d) nontoxigenic
3. *Vibrio mimicus*	(a) produces toxin similar to cholera toxin (b) produces a heat-stable toxin (c) nontoxigenic
4. *Vibrio parahaemolyticus*	(a) produces cardiotoxin (b) hemolytic (c) invasive
5. *Vibrio fluvialis* (EF-6)	(a) produces unique "toxin" (b) unknown mechanism
6. *Vibrio vulnificus*	unknown (invasive)
7. *Vibrio alginolyticus*	unknown (invasive)
8. *Vibrio metschnikovii*	unknown
9. *Vibrio hollisae*	unknown

routine use, do not detect toxins in many bacterial enteric pathogens isolated from disease, and incriminated epidemiologically. Organisms such as *V. fluvialis* (formerly called group EF-6 or group F) and classical EPEC strains are among these potentially important toxin-producing pathogens which would be missed by screens for traditional extracellular CT, LT, or ST. (e) Many of the assay systems described here require either sophisticated or expensive equipment, some technical expertise, and reagents which are often difficult to acquire (43).

There are both clinical and public health needs for at least some of these enterotoxin assays, but those needs may best be met at the reference laboratory level. Given the current commercial and research interests and efforts in the field of genetic engineering, the genetic probes may be modified to use labels other than radioactive isotypes in the near future. If stable and safe probes are developed, they could be invaluable in both the research and clinical laboratory. Additionally, there are specific serotype identifications which are strongly indicative of pathogenicity, and the clinical laboratory could provide these to clinicians and epidemiologists as tentative and contingent on verification by the reference laboratories. The problem in this area is that specific O (or H) antisera necessary to meaningfully type such organisms as *V. cholerae* non 01, *V. mimicus, Y. enterocolitica* or *E. coli* are not commercially available. However, our knowledge and expertise is increasing rapidly, providing sensitive and specific assays for the research and reference laboratories which, in turn, provide clinical and public health services.

REFERENCES

1. Bramucci, M. G. and R. K. Holmes. 1978. Radial passive immune hemolysis assay for detection of heat-labile enterotoxin produced by individual colonies of *Escherichia coli* or *Vibrio cholerae*. J. Clin. Microbiol. 8:252-255.

2. Brill, B. M., B. L. Wasilauskas, and S. H. Richardson. 1979. Adaptation of the staphylococcal coagglutination technique for detection of heat-labile enterotoxin of *Escherichia coli*. J. Clin. Microbiol. 9:49-55.

3. Burrows, W., and G. M. Musteikis. 1966. Cholera infection and toxin in the rabbit ileal loop. J. Infect. Dis. 116:183.

4. Craig, J. P. 1965. A permeability factor (toxin) found in cholera stools and culture filtrates and its neutralization by convalescent cholera sera. Nature 207:614-616.

5. Davis, B. R., G. R. Fanning, J. M. Madden, A. G. Steigerwalt, H. B. Bradford, H. L. Smith, and D. J. Brenner. 1981. Characterization of biochemically atypical *Vibrio cholerae* strains and designation of a new pathogenic species, *Vibrio mimicus*. J. Clin. Microbiol. 14:631-639.

6. Dean, A. G., J. C. Ching, R. G. Williams, and L. B. Harden. 1972. Test for *Escherichia coli* enterotoxin using infant mice: Application in a study of diarrhea in children in Honolulu. J. Infect. Dis. 125:407-411.

7. DeBoy, J. M., I, K. Wachsmuth, and B. Davis. 1980. Serotypes of enterotoxigenic *Escherichia coli* (ETEC) isolated in the United States. Infect. Immun. 29:361-368.

8. Donta, S. T., and M. King. 1973. Induction of steroidogenesis in tissue culture by cholera enterotoxin. Nature N. Biol. 243:246-247.

9. DuPont, H. L., S. B. Formal, and R. B. Hornick. 1971. Pathogenesis of *Escherichia coli* diarrhea. N. Engl. J. Med. 285:1-9.

10. Dutta, N. K., and M. K. Habbu. 1955. Experimental cholera in infant rabbits: Method for chemotherapeutic investigation. Brit. J. Pharmacol. 10:153.

11. Evans, D. G., D. J. Evans, W. S. Tjoa, and H. L. DuPont. 1978. Detection and characterization of colonization factor of enterotoxigenic *Escherichia coli* isolated from adults with diarrhea. Infect. Immun. 19:727-736.

12. Evans, D. J., D. G. Evans, H. L. DuPont, F. Orskov, and I. Orskov. 1977. Patterns of loss of enterotoxigenicity by *Escherichia coli* isolated from adults with diarrhea: Suggestive evidence for an interrelationship with serotype. Infect. Immun. 17:105-111.

13. Finkelstein, R. A. 1973. Cholera. CRC Crit. Rev. Microbiol. 2:553-623.

14. Gorbach, S. L., and C. M. Khurana. 1972. Toxigenic *Escherichia coli:* A cause of infantile diarrhea in Chicago. N. Engl. J. Med. 287:791-795.

15. Greenberg, H. B., D. A. Sack, W. Rodriguez, R. B. Sack, R. G. Wyatt, A. R. Kalica, R. L. Horswood, R. M. Chanock, and A. Z. Kapikian. 1977. Microtiter solid-phase radioimmunoassay for detection of *Escherichia coli* heat-labile enterotoxin. Infect. Immun. 17:541-545.

16. Guerrant, R. L., L. L. Brunton, T. C. Schnaitman, L. I. Robhun, and A. G. Gilman. 1974. Cyclic adenosine monophosphate and alteration of Chinese hamster ovary cell morphology: A rapid, sensitive *in vitro* assay for enterotoxins of *Vibrio cholerae* and *Escherichia coli*. Infect. Immun. 10:320-327.

17. Guerrant, R. L., M. D. Dickins, R. P. Wenzel, and A. Z. Kapikian. 1976. Toxigenic bacterial diarrhea: A nursery outbreak involving multiple bacterial strains. J. Pediat. 89:885-891.

18. Gyles, C. L., M. So, and S. Falkow. 1974. The enterotoxin plasmids of *Escherichia coli*. J. Infect. Dis. 130:40-49.

19. Hughes, J. M., J. M. Boyce, A. R. M. A. Aleem, J. G. Wells, A. S. M. Rahman, and G. T. Curlin. 1978. *Vibrio parahaemolyticus* enterocolitis in Bangladesh: Report of an outbreak. Am. J. Trop. Med. Hyg. 27:106-112.

20. Hughes, J. M., F. Murad, B. Chang, and R. L. Guerrant. 1978. Role of cyclic GMP in the action of heat-stable enterotoxin of *Escherichia coli*. Nature 271:755-756.

21. Kaper, J. B., S. L. Moseley, and S. Falkow. 1981. Molecular characterization of environmental and nontoxigenic strains of *Vibrio cholerae*. Infect. Immun. 32:661-667.

22. Keusch, G. T., and S. T. Donta. 1975. Classification of enterotoxins on the basis of activity in cell culture. J. Infact. Dis. 131:58-63.

23. Keusch, G. T., J. McIver, and G. F. Grady. 1975. Production and characterization of exotoxin(s) of *Shigella dysenteriae* Type 1. J. Infect. Dis. 131:559-566.

24. Klipstein, F. A., R. L. Guerrant, J. G. Wells, H. B. Short, and R. F. Engert. 1979. Comparison of assay of coliform enterotoxins by conventional techniques versus in vivo intestinal perfusion. Infect. Immun. 25:146-152.

25. Kusama, H., and J. P. Craig. 1970. Production of biologically active substances by two strains of *Vibrio cholerae*. Infect. Immun. 1:80-87.

26. Levine, M. M., E. J. Berquist, D. R. Nalin, D. H. Waterman, R. B. Hornick, C. R. Young, S. Sotman, and B. Rowe. 1978. *Escherichia coli* strains that cause diarrhea but do not produce heat-labile or heat-stable enterotoxins and are not invasive. The Lancet, May 27:1119-1122.

27. Ljungh, A., M. Popoff, and T. Wadstrom. 1977. *Aeromonas hydrophila* in acute diarrheal disease: Detection of enterotoxin and biotyping of strains. J. Clin. Microbiol. 6:96-100.

28. Lockwood, D. E., A. S. Kreger, and S. H. Richardson. 1982. Detection of toxins produced by *Vibrio fluvialis*. Infect. Immun. 35:702-708.

29. Morris, G. K., M. H. Merson, D. A. Sack, J. G. Wells, W. T. Martin, W. E. DeWitt, J. C. Feeley, R. B. Sack, and D. M. Bessudo. 1976. Laboratory investigation of diarrhea in travelers to Mexico: Evaluation of methods for detecting enterotoxigenic *Escherichia coli*. J. Clin. Microbiol. 3:486-495.

30. Moseley, S. L., I. Huq, A. R. M. A. Alim, M. So, M. Samadpour-Motalebi, and S. Falkow. 1981. Detection of enterotoxigenic *Escherichia coli* by DNA colony hybridization. J. Infect. Dis. 142:892-898.

31. Moseley, S. L., and S. Falkow. 1980. Nucleotide sequence homology between heat-labile enterotoxin gene of *Escherichia coli* and *Vibrio cholerae* deoxyribonucleic acid. J. Bacteriol. 144:444-446.

32. Orskov, I., and F. Orskov. 1977. Special O:K:H serotypes among enterotoxigenic *Escherichia coli* strains from diarrhea in adults and children. Med. Microbiol. Immunol. 163:99-110.

33. Rao, M. C., S. A. Orellana, M. Field, D. C. Robertson, and R. A. Gianella. 1981. Comparison of the biological actions of three purified heat-stable enterotoxins: Effects on ion transport and guanylate cyclase activity in the rabbit ileum in vitro. Infect. Immun. 33:165-170.

34. Rosenberg, M. L., J. P. Koplan, I. K. Wachsmuth, J. G. Wells, E. J. Gangarosa, R. L. Guerrant, and D. A. Sack. 1977. Epidemic diarrhea at Crater Lake: A large waterborne outbreak caused by enterotoxigenic *Escherichia coli*. Ann. Intern. Med. 86:714-718.

35. Ryder, R. W., I. K. Wachsmuth, A. E. Buxton, D. G. Evans, H. L. DuPont, E. Mason, and F. F. Barrett. 1976. Infantile diarrhea produced by heat-stable enterotoxigenic *Escherichia coli*. N. Engl. J. Med. 295:849-853.

36. Sack, D. A., and R. B. Sack. 1975. Test for enterotoxigenic *Escherichia coli* using Y1 adrenal cells in miniculture. Infect. Immun. 11:334-336.

37. Sack. R. B. 1975. Human diarrheal disease caused by enterotoxigenic *Escherichia coli*. Ann. Rev. Microbiol. 29:333-353.

38. Sandefur, P. D., and J. W. Peterson. 1977. Neutralization of *Salmonella* toxin-induced elongation of Chinese hamster ovary cells by cholera antitoxin. Infect. Immun. 15:988-992.

39. So, M., F. Heffron, and B. J. McCarthy. 1979. The *E. coli* gene encoding heat-stable toxin is a bacterial transposon flanked by inverted repeats of IS1. Nature 277:453-456.

40. Southern, E. M. 1975. Detection of specific sequences among DNA fragments separated by gel electrophoresis. J. Mol. Biol. 98:503-517.

41. Spira, W. M., R. B. Sack, and J. L. Froehlich. 1981. Simple adult rabbit model for *Vibrio cholerae* and enterotoxigenic *Escherichia coli* diarrhea. Infect. Immun. 32:739-747.

42. Svennerholm, A., and J. Holmgren. 1978. Identification of *Escherichia coli* heat-labile enterotoxin by means of a ganglioside immunosorbent assay (G_{M1}-ELISA) procedure. Curr. Microbiol. 1:19-23.

43. Wachsmuth, I. K. 1980. *Escherichia coli* typing and pathogenicity. Clin. Microbiol. Newsletter 2(12):4-7.

44. Wachsmuth, I. K., S. Falkow, and Ryder, R. W. 1976. Plasmid-mediated properties of an enterotoxigenic *Escherichia coli* associated with infantile diarrhea. Infect. Immun. 14:403-407.

45. Wachsmuth, I. K., J. G. Wells, P. Shipley, and R. W. Ryder. 1979. Heat-labile enterotoxin production in isolates from a shipboard outbreak of human diarrheal illness. Infect. Immun. 24:793-797.

46. Yolken, R. H., H. B. Greenberg, M. H. Merson, R. B. Sack, and A. Z. Kapikian. 1977. Enzyme-linked immunosorbent assay for detection of *Escherichia coli* heat-labile enterotoxin. J. Clin. Microbiol. 6:439-444.

7

Amebiasis and Giardiasis

JOHN D. FRAME
Division of Tropical Medicine
School of Public Health
Columbia University
College of Physicians and Surgeons
New York, New York

I. AMEBIASIS

Entamoeba histolytica Schaudinn, 1903, is the cause of human intestinal amebiasis; occasional instances of infection with *E. polecki* von Prowazek, 1912 have been reported (1,2). *Dientameba fragilis* Jepps and Dobell, 1918, another agent of diarrheal disease, is now considered to be a flagellate (3).

Not all persons are symptomatic in whom organisms are found which are structurally identical with *E. histolytica*. It has been postulated that *E. histolytica* is a pathogen living as a commensal in many individual patients (4.5). Recent work, however, suggests that there are biochemical differences between commensal and pathogenic forms (see below). Differences in the sizes of otherwise morphologically similar organisms have been noted, and the small organisms are now generally classified as *E. hartmanni* von Prowazek, 1912 (6), a nonpathogen. Neal (7) pointed out that though under varying cultural conditions in the laboratory *E. histolytica* strains will change size, under comparable circumstances there is a bimodal distribution of organisms that are structurally similar. He summarized the results of previous investigations showing that though there may be slight overlap in size, the difference of the average diameters of cysts of the two groups is about 4 - 5μ.

Clinical laboratories have in general only recently taken cognizance of the differences between *E. histolytica* and *E. hartmanni*. Other fruits of research are likely soon to be exploited in the laboratory diagnosis of amebiasis. Some of them as well as the usual clinical parasitological topics are reviewed in this chapter.

A. Classification

On the basis of clinical-pathological considerations, cultural requirements, and biochemical and serological tests three major categories of *Entamoebae* infecting humans may be described which are morphologically indistinguishable except for size:

Large -- average cyst diameter more than 10 microns
E. histolytica -- pathogenic and nonpathogenic, *E. histolytica-like* -- nonpathogenic (8)

Small -- average cyst diameter less than 10 microns,
E. hartmanni -- nonpathogenic

The term "*E. histolytica*-like" is applied to a group of amebae which differ from pathogenic *E. histolytica* in a number of characteristics. Beaver, Jung, Sherman, Read and Robinson, (9,10) testing experimental infection of volunteers used a strain (later designated as "Huff") from an asymptomatic cyst passer. No recipient developed dysentery, and diarrhea was more common in controls than in the infected group. Under experimental conditions the organism caused characteristic ulcerations in dogs, guinea pigs and rats with frequences comparable to those in animals inoculated with a strain isolated from a child who had severe dysentery.

The "Laredo" strain (11) was obtained from a patient with diarrhea whose symptoms disappeared with removal of a colonic polyp. It could be cultured at room as well as body temperature (12) and was ten times as resistant to emetine as the usual strains of *E. histolytica* (13).

The JA and AG strains were obtained from asymptomatic cyst passers (14,15). They were able to grow at room temperature and at 37°C, and were ten times as resistant to emetine as the K-9 strain, isolated from a symptomatic patient (15).

Strain "403" (16) was derived from an asymptomatic cyst carrier. It was grown at both 27° and 35°C. This strain and the previous four multiplied in hypotonic solutions to a dilution of 1:32, and then encysted; in contrast, eight strains derived from symptomatic patients did not survive dilutions of 1:4 (16).

Differences between the *E. histolytica*-like strains and known pathogenic *E. histolytica* have also been noted by tests with fluorescent antibody (11,17,18), and growth characteristics in a CO_2-bicarbonate buffer system (14). Goldman (18) has discussed these and other differences in detail.

The clearest demonstration of a biochemical basis for the classification of the structurally similar strains of the *E. histolytica* group derives from the experiments of Sargeaunt, Williams and their colleagues. They conducted a number of investigations of the isoenzymes of amebae by the thin-layer starch-gel electrophoresis method of Wraxall and Culliford (19). Using the cultures grown by the method of Robinson (20), in which the organisms are grown in the presence of intestinal bacteria, they studied malate oxidoreductase (ME), glucose-phosphate isomerase (GPI), phosphoglucomutase (PGM) (21) and later, hexokinase (HK) (22) in strains of amebae from their own laboratories, various hospitals in the United Kingdom and from India. They found differences between the isoenzyme patterns of *E. histolytica* and *E. coli*, a commensal (21). Among the former they were able to classify four isoenzyme groups, and to distinguish the strains from symptomatic and asymptomatic patients on the basis of PGM and GPI (21,23). *E. hartmanni* showed a distinctive enzyme pattern (23). The *E. histolytica*-like organisms formed a single isoenzyme group differing from any of the *E. histolytica* patterns (24). Isoenzyme patterns of strains identified as *E. polecki* resembled those of the various nonpathogenic *E. histolytica* groups (24).

Extending their work to Mexico City, they isolated 125 organisms from patients seen in various hospitals there (25). They distinguished 11 groups of *E. histolytica* as well as strains of *E. coli*, *E. hartmanni*, *D. fragilis* and *Iodamoeba buetschlii*. Patients with clinical amebiasis fell into three groups of varied isoenzyme patterns; they shared a single PGM line in the β position, and a slow moving HK line. Some groups of strains from carriers with both β and β PGM lines could be distinguished from the pathogenic strains by a rapidly moving HK line characteristic of nonpathogenic strains.

If the results of isoenzyme electrophoresis are confirmed, the technique may become required for the clinical laboratory diagnosis of pathogenic amebae.

B. Pathogenicity

When an organism identified as *E. histolytica* is found in a stool specimen, the question of its pathogenicity confronts the clinician and clinical pathologist. The decision is generally easy in the case of acute dysentery or liver abscess, but not so in a mildly symptomatic or asymptomatic patient. The organism may not be the cause of the symptoms in the first instance. In the second, the issue is whether the host is a carrier who may become the cause of disease in someone infected by him. It would be helpful if there were means of determining the virulence of the discovered organism.

Experiments on virulence of *E. histolytica* have been performed in the main with animals which are not its natural host. Under these circumstances some normally pathogenic amebae are found to lose virulence after several passages in axenic culture, and regain it after repeated colonic passage (26), by multiple hamster liver passages (27), by alternating liver and monoxenic passages (28) and by axenic culture in the presence of cholesterol (29). On the other hand, there is a limit to the enhancement of virulence by these manipulations; it is apparently difficult to establish a reproducible animal model for the investigation of tissue invasion by *E. histolytica* (30). Furthermore, the relevance of the laboratory finding to clinical amebiasis is unclear.

In a series of experiments the virulence of amebic strains obtained from patients was tested in the brain of the newborn mouse (31), the new-born hamster (32) and baby hamster kidney cells (33). There was general congruence in the results of the assays in different models, but there were some exceptions, the most notable the strain HK-9. The organism was classified as avirulent in the mouse brain, slightly virulent in the newborn hamster, and among the most virulent of strains when tested in cell culture.

In another assay the hemolytic activity of total homogenate of trophozoites of several strains of amebae was tested against mammalian erythrocytes (34). Of three strains of *E. histolytica*, HK-9 and HM-2:IMSS showed low, and HM-3:IMSS, moderate activity against human erythrocytes; in general, all three showed stronger reactions to non-human erythrocytes. The relative activity of the strains was the reverse of the results in newborn hamster and hamster kidney cell assays (32,33). The Laredo *E. histolytica*-like strain showed no hemolytic activity with human cells, but a little against two of the other six mammalian red blood cells.

Neal, Robinson, Lewis and Kessel (4) compared the clinical findings of patients infected with *E. histolytica* with indirect hemagglutination (IHA) titers of the sera, and the virulence of their amebae injected into rat ceca. Seven symptomatic patients gave high IHA titers on serological testing; their amebae were also virulent to rats, though the degree of virulence of one strain was low. There was good correlation in the whole group of 40 between the "cecal scores" in rats, and the IHA titers of the patients from whom the strains had been isolated.

That isolates from acutely ill amebic patients could infect and produce ulcers in significantly more rats than isolates from asymptotmatic cyst passers was subsequently confirmed (35). However, it was concluded that serological titers showed minimal or no correlation with the severity of the disease.

The isoenzyme electrophoretic technique of Sargeaunt and his co-workers (25), if confirmed by testing on other populations, appears to be the most likely candidate to become a means to determine the pathogenicity of *E. histolytica* in the clinical laboratory.

C. Culture

The culture of *E. histolytica* from stool and abscess specimens, long used in the experimental laboratory, is being carried out in some diagnostic laboratories as well. The method is based on that of Robinson (20), with cultivation of amebae in the presence of the flora of the original specimens.

Axenic culture by the method of Diamond (36) is used in experimental situations, the medium has been modified by Diamond, Harlow and Cunnick (37). In the latter technique smaller inocula of amebae were required to establish cultures, yields were greater, growth more uniform, and in the case of *E. histolytica*, generation time was reduced one third.

A method for the cultivation of amebae from small inocula has been described (38), as well as techniques for the separation of clonal cultures (39,40).

D. Microscopic Examination

Microscopic examination of stool, proctosigmoidoscopic material or abscess contents remains the only means for the indisputable diagnosis of infection with *E. histolytica* (41). However, the diagnosis is often missed in the clinical laboratory. In the best of laboratories the parasites will be found in no more than 70% of specimens in a single examination. Amebae will be discovered in the stool in about 12 to 15% of cases of amebic liver abscess at the time the abscess is diagnosed.

Evaluation of the errors in microscopic examination show that overdiagnosis results from confusion with polymorphonuclear leukocytes, or with nonpathogenic amebae, and underdiagnosis by mishandling of the specimen and nonrecognition of the parasites (41).

The specimen must be examined while it is fresh; if this is not possible, it should be stored at 4°C. to prevent lysis of the organism. A methylene blue diluent will help distinguish amebae from leukocytes. Specimens may also be fixed while fresh with polyvinyl alcohol (PVA) or Schaudinn's preservative, and stained with Wheatley-Gomori trichrome stain (42). Among 41 laboratory workers attending a training workshop in parasitology, *Entamoeba* trophozoites were recognized 4.8% of the time in freshmount specimens, and 58.5% of the time in PVA preserved and stained specimens (43). Calibrated ocular micrometers are essential to permit differentiation of *E. histolytica* from *E. hartmanni* (41).

Specimens mixed with PVA by the patient immediately after collection will permit diagnosis more frequently than those brought to the laboratory and preserved with Schaudinn's preservative there

(44). A two-bottle technique has been suggested, with formalin as a preservative in one-bottle and PVA in the other (45). Another two-vial technique with one empty bottle and one with Schaudinn's fluid was tested (46); the unpreserved specimen revealed 20% fewer stools positive for protozoa than the preserved. However, helminths were diagnosed far more frequently in the unpreserved, suggesting the value of the two-bottle technique for the clinical laboratory.

Material from proctosigmoidoscopy should be collected by curette, biopsy punch or glass aspirator; amebae tend to adhere to cotton swabs (41).

The direct immunofluorescent staining technique was the most sensitive for the detection of amebae in ethanol-fixed rectal biopsies (47). The PAS stain was almost as efficient. The indirect immunofluorescent technique was more sensitive than conventional stains with formalin fixed tissues. At best, 15% of aspirate positive dysentery patients are negative on biopsy of colonic mucosa.

E. Immunodiagnosis

The indirect hemagglutination (IHA) test has long set the standard for the epidemiological and clinical investigation of amebiasis (48). However, amebic antibodies as found by IHA persist, albeit with slowly falling titers, long after clinical recovery of the patient (49). About 97% of patients with amebic liver abscess, and 90% with amebic dysentery will be positive, as well as 40% of symptomless cyst passers.

Various precipitin tests are also in use. The double diffusion Ouchterlony technique compared well with IHA (50,51); the original method required four days for completion. This gel diffusion precipitin (GDP) test has been modified by others; as described by Patterson, Healy and Shabot (52), the test may be completed in 24 to 48 hours. It apparently detects a different antibody than does IHA (51,52). Antibodies persist for some time after the patient's clinical cure.

The cellulose acetate membrane precipitin (CAP) test (53) is performed in a moist chamber with strips of cellulose acetate membrane replacing conventional agar gel. It is possible to place antigen in the center well, dry the membrane and store it for future use in the field; the membrane, moistened with buffer is reconstituted for use. The test is apparently faster than the GDP, requiring four and one-half hours for completion, and the results are comparable. In one experiment comparison of the CAP results with the presence of immunoglobulins by indirect immunofluorescence (54) consistently showed raised anti-amebic IgG in patients in whom the precipitin test was positive. No relationship was found between the presence of amebaspecific IgM or IgA and the results of the test.

Counterimmunoelectrophoresis (CIEP) (55) compares favorably with IHA, and is more sensitive than GDP (56). The test is faster than the standard diffusion tests, and in this compares with the time required for IFA. Valuable in the clinical laboratory, it has limited application for field use because of the need for reliable electric power and special equipment.

Thin layer immunoassay (TIA) has been suggested as a test that because of technical simplicity and low cost may be used for screening patient sera for antibodies to *Entamoeba histolytica* (57). Polystyrene petri dishes are coated with an aqueous solution of *E. histolytica* antigen, agar poured into the plates and holes for the sera to be tested punched in the congealed agar. The areas of reaction are measured to give quantitative as well as qualitative results. Further evaluation of the test is needed to determine its specificity and range of usefulness.

Indirect immunofluorescence (IIF) is being used widely for the diagnosis of amebiasis in the clinical laboratory (58). In a large series in France it was found positive in all cases of amebic liver abscess, 59% of cases of amebic dysentery, 31% of amebic colitis and 21% of "post-amebic colitis"; it was also positive in 15% of cyst passers (59). If a titer of 1:50 was taken as a threshold for specificity, none of 1,217 sera from patients without amebiasis were positive. In treated amebic abscess of the liver titers showed a distinct fall about three weeks after completion of treatment -- aspiration of the abscess together with chemotherapy. In the field, IIF has been found sensitive, specific and reproducible. Ninety-six percent of amebic liver abscess patients, 73% of those with amebic dysentery, 15% of amebic colitis and 9% of asymptomatic amebiasis were found positive, whereas no positive sera were found above a titer of 1:16 among 25 healthy subjects (60).

Enzyme linked immunosorbent assay (ELISA) has been performed with horseradish peroxidase (61,62,63) and alkaline phosphatase (64,65) conjugates. In field tests (66) ELISA was found practical, to be more sensitive than GDP and CIEP and more rapid than the former. The fact that it does not require electrical power and equipment gives the ELISA another advantage over CIEP. Testing of the serological response of experimentally infected golden hamsters showed ELISA to be as sensitive as IHA (62). The development of a standardized ELISA suitable for the clinical laboratory has been reported (65). Comparison of ELISA with IHA (67) showed good congruence in the diagnosis of amebic liver abscess, and more sensitivity in intestinal amebiasis. In patients with "non-specific hepatomegaly" ELISA was positive while stool examination and IHA were negative. No follow-up was reported, so that it was not clear whether these results indicated superior sensitivity or inferior specificity.

On the basis of their experience with ELISA reactions in plague, Williams and Robinson (68) have suggested that the use of ELISA-inhibition controls is appropriate as a means of testing for non-specific responses in other applications of the test. They added small amounts of antigen to the serum diluent to accomplish this end.

ELISA with peroxidase-labeled IgG antibody has also been used for the detection of *E. histolytica* antigen in fecal samples (69). Of 1177 single fecal samples tested, 155 were positive by both microscopic examination and ELISA, four by microscopic examination only and 255 by ELISA only. In another experiment with 382 specimens from 155 patients, 52 patients were positive by boty microscopy and ELISA and 60 by ELISA only (70). Eighty-five stool specimens for a number of other intestinal protozoa and helminths were negative by *E. histolytica* by ELISA (69). Confirmation of these results is required to determine the significance of the large numbers of specimens positive by ELISA and negative by microscopic examination. The finding is possibly due to the presence of very small numbers of intact organisms amenable to microscopic examination (70). Stool cultures and longitudinal studies will likely be used to test this hypothesis, and an alternate possibility that ELISA detects fecal antigen persisting after treatment and cure of the patients.

Radio-immunoassay (RIA) shows sensitivity comparable to that of ELISA in the diagnosis of amebic liver abscess (71), but the need for special equipment renders it impractical for field work.

In summary, serological tests are very useful in the diagnosis of liver abacess, and almost as valuable in the case of amebic dysentery. Some comments from the Centers for Disease Control regarding the diagnosis of invasive amebiasis are illuminating:

> "In our experience, the fecal examination had a sensitivity of 0.387, the GDP test, 0.914, and the IHA test, 0.935. The specificity of the fecal examination is 0.979, the GDP test, 0.991, and the IHA test, 0.946. The positive predictive value of fecal examination is 0.900, the GDP test, 0.941, and the IHA test, 0.707. The negative predictive value of fecal examination is 0.881, the GDP test, 0.987, and the IHA test, 0.991.
>
> "All methods are highly specific; however, the fecal examination is quite insensitive, while the IHA test is the most sensitive. The GDP test is clearly superior in terms of positive predictive value. The GDP test and the IHA test are both superior in terms of negative predictive value." (52).

The significance of the relatively low sensitivity of the serological tests of persons with "luminal" infection or in the "carrier state" cannot be evaluated until the actual or potential pathogenicity of the organisms that infect them have been evaluated by investigations such as those reviewed earlier in this chapter.

II. GIARDIASIS

Giardia lamblia Stiles, 1915 is the parasitic agent of giardiasis, a gastrointestinal disorder of varied symptomatology. It is the intestinal parasite most frequently identified in public health laboratories in the United States (72). The presence of the protozoa in the jejunum may cause no symptoms at all, a state demonstrated by infection studies in which only one of 21 persons infected by cysts from a carrier complained of gastrointestinal symptoms; this patient had similar complaints when no parasites could be found in his stool (73). Epigastric discomfort, anorexia, abdominal pain, per--sistant mild to severe diarrhea, steatorrhea and malabsorption syndrome with weight loss and fatigue may occur (74). Though at times it may not be certain that a patient's symptoms are in fact due to the *Giardia* discovered in his stool, at present it is generally accepted that *G. lamblia* infection is in fact a cause of diarrheal disease (73), and should be considered in patients with a medical history of diarrhea or malabsorption.

A. Classification

Mammalian *Giardia* are at present suspected of including two species, *G. muris* in rodents and *G. duodenalis* infecting a wide range of warm-blooded vertebrates (75,76). The issue has not been resolved, and until it has been, the traditional name *G. lamblia* appears to continue appropriate for the American clinician, in Europe the organism is called *G. intestinalis* and in East Europe, *Lamblia intestinalis* (77).

B. Culture

At present culture of *G. lamblia* appears to be significant for the clinical pathologist primarily for the procuring of antigen for serological tests.

An earlier technique for the axenic culture of *Giardia* in a medium containing 15-20% human serum (78) was found to produce erratic results by Visvesvara, who then adapted (79) the medium of Diamond (36). Another technique has been described for the clonal growth of *Giardia* on an agarose medium (80). If inocula were diluted to permit the growth of only a few colonies per plate, they could be removed and established satisfactorily in liquid medium.

Cryopreservation of trophozoites has been described (81). After freezing and storing in liquid nitrogen, incubation at 37°C allowed recovery with more than 50% motility of the organisms.

A method for the pure preparation of cysts from stools (82) has been reported requiring initial concentration by the formal ether technique, separation by centrifugation in a density gradient, and filtration through a nucleopore filter.

C. Microscopic Diagnosis

Trophozoites or cysts may be diagnosed in the stool and trophozoites in jejunal biopsy, duodenal lavage or by means of a braided nylon string swallowed in a capsule (Enterotest, Hedeco, Palo Alto, California). In the examination of stools passed by children over periods of one to three months three patterns of excretion were observed (83). *High* secretors with parasites in nearly all stools, *low* with scanty numbers present in about 40% of stools, and *mixed* with periods of high secretion for periods of one to three weeks alternating with a generally shorter period of low excretion. The overall frequency of positive stools was about 60%. The presence and relative numbers of *Giardia* in the feces did not seem to be related to either consistency of the stools or frequency of defecation. In general, purgation was not successful in increasing parasite excretion. In one mixed excretor the stools were negative for *Giardia* for 20 consecutive days, before they became positive again.

The authors found no appreciable change in the number of trophozoites or cysts if the stools were stored at 4°C. for 48 hours, and felt there was no need for chemical preservation. Other investigators have noted among specimens mailed to the laboratory 28% more stools positive for *Giardia* when they were preserved in Schaudinn's fixative than when unpreserved stools were returned (47). In yet another study, equal numbers of *Giardia* were found in specimens preserved by the patient in polyvinyl alcohol, and those brought to the laboratory within four hours and fixed there in Schaudinn's fixative (45). A few specimens in which one or the other was positive and the alternative technique negative revealed very low cyst counts, and differences were ascribed to observational chance.

Nylon yarn coiled within a weighted gelatin capsule and swallowed by the patient may be used to sample duodenal contents (84). In one small series of six patients, the nylon yarn recovered *Giardia* trophozoites in 5, the Crosby capsule by jejunal biopsy 4, and stool examination, four with cysts, two positive in each of two examinations (85). It is reported that only infrequently is this test or duodenal aspiration negative when a stool examination is positive (86). But Wolfe (87) stated that he rarely found the technique positive in the face of negative stool examinations.

In a comparative study of four techniques (88), a combination of stool examination, duodenal aspiration, mucosal impression smears of biopsy specimens and microscopic examinations of the specimens disclosed 12 patients positive for giardiasis. Stool examination was positive in six, and duodenal aspiration in 10; combined results were diagnostic in all twelve. Both histological examination and smear preparations of the biopsies were positive in 12. Detection of the parasites by histological techniques was time-consuming, and the impression smear was recommended as a useful initial step in the routine evaluation of intestinal biopsies.

D. Serodiagnosis

A complement fixation technique for the detection of serum antibodies in *Giardia* was described previously (89). More recently, the indirect immunofluorescent test (IIF) with cyst antigen demonstrated a crude correlation between the antibody titer and the severity of the histopathological lesion in the jejunum (90). However, it was difficult to obtain reliable antigen; of the samples tested as antigen, two liquid stools containing thin-walled precysts were suitable, and mature cysts did not give completely reproducible results. In another investigation with this technique IIF was positive in 18 out of 19 cases of giardiasis with malabsorption, and negative in patients with gluten enteropathy and inflammatory bowel disease and in 10 of 11 patients with acute topical sprue (91).

Subsequently, IIF with the use of trophozoites cultured axenically was described (92). Specificity of the antibodies was demonstrated by absorption with *G. lamblia*, but not with *E. histolytica*, *Trichomonas vaginalis* or *Escherichia coli*. Giardiasis patients with hypogammaglobulinemia had no detectable antibody against *G. lamblia*.

IIF with a cyst antigen prepared on a ficol-urographin density gradient (82) was found to have a higher rate of positivity than indirect hemagglutination (IHA) using a trophozoite antigen (93), but a predominance of precyst stages of *Giardia* appeared to be necessary for effective testing. IHA required no costly equipment and the antigen could be stored; it was preferred by the investigators for these reasons. Mice fed with cysts of *G. lamblia* (94) were used to obtain trophozoites used in the IHA antigen.

Immunodiffusion by an Ouchterlony technique revealed precipitins in the sera of 10 of 11 patients with giardiasis as demonstrated by stool examination and duodenal aspirate (95). Antigen was from cysts obtained by flotation in 33% zinc sulphate which were then sonicated, and centrifuged cold, with the supernatant being used.

The keeping quality of the antigen was poor, and only two of seven batches were satisfactorily in the gel tests.

An ELISA using alkaline-phosphatase-labeled goat antihuman-IgG globulin and unfixed intact *G. lamblia* trophozoites was found to be sensitive and reproducible (86). Eighty-one percent of 59 symptomatic giardiasis patients had detectable antibody, as did 14% of uninfected controls. Optical density (OD) was used as the endpoint. At higher dilutions reduction of the OD to background levels by *G. lamblia* but not with *T. vaginalis* or *E. histolytica* demonstrated the specificity of the test. Antibody may be present for at least 15 months after infection. OD readings were higher with intact than with sonicated organisms, suggesting that the IgG anti-*G. lamblia* antibodies are directed against surface antigens or products of secretion or excretion.

III. SEXUALLY TRANSMITTED PROTOZOAL DIARRHEAS

The possibility of sexual transmission of protozoa has been suggested in the past (96,97). Shookhoff (98) and Lynch (99), responding to previous correspondence regarding a patient infected with *G. lamblia, D. fragilis* and other intestinal parasites (100) believed anal-oral contact had been the means of infection. Numerous publications have by now implicated homosexual practices in infections with *E. histolytica* (101,102), *G. lamblia* (103) and *D. fragilis* (104). *Cryptosporidium*, a parasite of veterinary importance, has recently been reported in homosexuals (105,106). It will be discussed below.

Ano-oral sexual contact is the apparent route of infection of sexually acquired amebiasis and giardiasis, both among heterosexuals and homosexuals (101,103,107). However, most cases of sexually transmitted protozoal infections are found among homosexuals, presumably because of their common practice of analingus and fellatio, and a high degree of sexual activity with numerous partners (104).

A significant problem in the management of parasitized homosexuals is the issue of recurrent illness (101). One possible cause is reinfection, and recurring infection has been stopped by change of sexual practices (107). It is also possible that the initial or subsequent diagnosis was erroneous. Leukocytes or *E. hartmanni* not adequately differentiated from *E. histolytica* by its smaller size may have been the organisms seen by the parasitic technologist. At times other infectious agents cause persistent symptoms; treatment of shigellosis has lead to cure of what was clinically considered to be recurring amebiasis (108).

Treatment failure because of drug resistance must also be considered as a cause of recurrent infection. Metronidazole is known to be highly effective in the treatment of intestinal amebiasis and giardiasis, and quinacrine in giardiasis. However, even in carefully observed cases treatment failure does appear to be more frequent among homosexuals than the experience of the parasitologist would lead him to expect (101).

The possibility that the symptoms of the patient may be due to some other agent of the "Gay Bowel Syndrome" (109), and not to amebae found on stool examination must be considered. Appropriate laboratory evaluation of possible cases of sexually transmitted protozoal infections may well include adequate cultures for bacterial infections as well as stool examination for intestinal parasites.

No investigation has been reported for the possible presence of *E. histolytica*-like organisms which in the past have been found resistant to some antiamebic drugs (13,15). Furthermore, the ameba may be essentially nonpathogenic. No relationship between infection with amebae and symptoms was found in a survey in which homosexual males mailed in specimens with a completed questionnaire, nor among firemen in a control group (110).

None of 22 homosexuals with stool-positive amebiasis at the time of examination or in the recent past have been found to have antibodies when tested by IHA at the Centers for Disease Control, Atlanta (111). In the past about 15% to 66% of cyst passers and over 90% of patients with mild to moderate symptoms have been found positive by workers investigating apparently non-venereal amebiasis (48,51).

Cryptosporidium sp. has been identified in six homosexual patients (105,106) in New York. Epidemiologic and information is still incomplete. Organisms are being identified by means of flotation by Sheather's technique (112) and by staining with a modified acid-fast stain to distinguish oocysts of *Cryptosporidium* from *Blastocystis hominis*, which does not stain by this technique.

Cryptosporidium has recently been identified in a presumably healthy young male free of immune deficiencies who had started a survey of calves for *Cryptosporidium* (113). Stool examinations of 16 other animals handlers at the institution identified 11 other cases of cryptosporidiosis (114). All but two were symptomatic with illnesses that lasted for relatively short periods of time, 14 days in the case of the initial patient.

Eight of 12 cases from the literature (114) were in people who were immunologically deficient or who were undergoing immunosuppressive therapy. The diarrhea tended to be prolonged in them. It remains to be demonstrated whether the recently reported cases among homosexuals are related to the acquired immunodeficiency disease of unknown etiology recently reported primarily among homosexual males (115).

REFERENCES

1. Levin, R. L., and Armstrong, D. E. *Am. J. Clin. Pathol., 54:*611 (1970).

2. Chacin-Bonilla, L. *Am. J. Trop. Med. Hyg., 29:*521 (1980).

3. Camp, R. R., Mattern, C. F. T., and Honigberg, B. M. *J. Protozool., 21:*69 (1974).

4. Neal, R. A., Robinson, G. L., Lewis, W. P., and Kessel, J. F. *Trans. Roy. Soc. Trop. Med. Hyg., 62:*69 (1968).

5. World Health Organization Expert Committee. *W.H.O. Tech. Rpt. Ser. No. 421,* p. 9 (1969).

6. Elsdon-Dew, R. *Advances in Parasitology, 6:*1 (1968).

7. Neal, R. A. in *Advances in Parasitology* (B. Dawes, ed.) Vol. 4, Academic Press, New York and London, 1966, p. 2.

8. World Health Organization Expert Committee, ibid. p. 22.

9. Beaver, P. C., Jung, R. C., Sherman, H. J., Read, T. R., and Robinson, T. A. *Am. J. Trop. Med. Hyg., 5:*1000 (1956).

10. Beaver, P. C., Jung, R. C., Sherman, H. J., Read, T. R., and Robinson, T. A. *Am. J. Trop. Med. Hyg., 5:*1015 (1956).

11. Goldman, M., Gleason, N. N., and Carver, R. K. *Amer. J. Trop. Med. Hyg., 11:*341 (1962).

12. Dreyer, D. A. *Texas Reports on Biol. and Med., 19:*393 (1961).

13. Entner, N., Evans, L. A., and Gonzales, C. *J. Protozool., 9:*466 (1962).

14. Nelson, E. C., and Jones, M. M. *Am. J. Trop. Med. Hyg., 13:* 667 (1964).

15. Entner, N., and Most, H. *J. Protozool., 12:*10 (1965).

16. Richards, C. S., Goldman, M., and Cannon, L. T. *Am. J. Trop. Med. Hyg., 15:*648 (1966).

17. Goldman, M., and Cannon, L. T. *Am. J. Trop. Med. Hyg., 16:*245 (1967).

18. Goldman, M. *Bull. W.H.O., 40:*355 (1969).

19. Wraxall, B. G. D., and Culliford, B. J. *J. Forensic Sci. Soc., 8:*81 (1968).

20. Robinson, G. L. *Trans. Roy. Soc. Trop. Med. Hyg., 62:*285 (1968).

21. Sargeaunt, P. G., and Williams, J. E. *Trans. Roy. Soc. Trop. Med. Hyg., 72:*164 (1978).

22. Farri, T. A., Sargeaunt, P. G., Warhurst, D. C., Williams, J. E., and Bhojnani, R. *Trans. Roy. Soc. Trop. Med. Hyg., 74:*672 (1980).

23. Sargeaunt, P. G., and Williams, J. E. *Trans. Roy. Soc. Trop. Med. Hyg., 73:*225 (1979).

24. Sargeaunt, P. G., Williams, J. E., and Neal, R. A. *Trans. Roy. Soc. Trop. Med. Hyg., 74:*469 (1980).

25. Sargeaunt, P. G., Williams, J. E., Kumate, J., and Jimenez, E. *Trans. Roy. Soc. Trop. Med. Hyg., 74:*653 (1980).

26. Thompson, P. E., McCarthy, D., and Reinertson, J. W. *Am. J. Hyg., 59:*249 (1954).

27. Lushbaugh, W. B., Kairalla, A. B., Loadholt, C. B., and Pittman, F. E. *Am. J. Trop. Med. Hyg., 27:*248 (1978).

28. Bos, H. J., and Hage, A. J. *Z. Parasitenk., 47:*79 (1975).

29. Bos, H. J., and Van de Griend, R. J. *Nature, 265:*341 (1977).

30. Gold, D., and Norman, L. *J. Parasitol. 65:*970 (1979).

31. Mattern, C. F. T., and Keister, D. B. *Am. J. Trop. Med. Hyg., 26:*393 (1977).

32. Mattern, C. F. T., and Keister, D. B. *Am. J. Trop. Med. Hyg., 26:*402 (1977).

33. Mattern, C. F. T., Keister, D. B., and Caspar, P. A. *Am. J. Trop. Med. Hyg., 27:*882 (1978).

34. Lopez-Revilla, R., and Said, F. *Am. J. Trop. Med. Hyg., 29:* 209 (1980).

35. Vinayak, V. K., Sawhney, R., Jain, P., Chugh, S., Naik, S. R., and Chakravarti, R. N. *Trans. Roy. Soc. Trop. Med. Hyg., 75:*32 (1981).

36. Diamond, L. S. *J. Parasitol., 54:*1047 (1968).

37. Diamond, L. S., Harlow, D. R., and Cunnick, C. C. *Trans. Roy. Soc. Trop. Med. Hyg., 72:*431 (1978).

38. Dutta, G. P. *India J. Med. Res., 54:*573 (1976).

39. Farri, T. A. *Trans. Roy. Soc. Trop. Med. Hyg., 72:*205 (1978).

40. Gillin, F. D., and Diamond, L. S. *J. Protozool., 25:*539 (1978).

41. Krogstad, D. J., Spencer, H. C., Healy, G. R., Gleason, N. N., Sexton, D. J., and Herron, C. A. *Ann. Int. Med., 88:*89 (1978).

42. Wheatley, W. B. *Am. J. Clin. Path., 21:*990 (1951).

43. Gardner, B. B., Del Junco, D. J., Fenn, J., and Hengesbaugh, J. H. *J. Clin. Microbiol., 12:*656 (1980).

44. Markell, E. K., and Quinn, P. M. *Am. J. Trop. Med. Hyg., 26:* 1139 (1977).

45. Brooke, M. M., and Goldman, M. *J. Lab. Clin. Med., 34:*1554 (1949).

46. Scholten, T. H., and Yang, J. *Am. J. Clin. Path., 62:*563 (1974).

47. Gilman, R., Islam, M., Paschi, S., Goleburn, J., and Ahmad, F. *Gastroenterology, 78:*435 (1980).

48. Kessel, J. F., Lewis, W. P., Pasquel, C. M., and Turner, J. A. *Am. J. Trop. Med. Hyg., 14:*540 (1965).

49. Milgram, E. A., Healy, G. R., and Kagan, I. G. *Gastroenterology, 50:*645 (1966).

50. Maddison, S. E., Powell, S. J., and Elsdon-Dew, R. *Am. J. Trop. Med. Hyg., 14:*554 (1965).

51. Maddison, S. E., Powell, S. J., and Elsdon-Dew, R. *Am. J. Trop. Med. Hyg., 14:*551 (1965).

52. Patterson, M., Healy, G. R., and Shabot, M. *Gastroenterology, 76:*136 (1980).

53. Stamm, W. P., and Phillips, E. A. *Trans. Roy. Soc. Trop. Med. Hyg., 71:*490 (1977).

54. Osisanya, J. O. S., and Warhurst, D. C. *Trans. Roy. Soc. Trop. Med. Hyg., 74:*605 (1980).

55. Sepulveda, B., Lee, E., Torre, M. de la, and Landa, L. *Arch. Invest. Med., 2*(Suppl): 263 (1971).

56. Krupp, Iris, M. *Am. J. Trop. Med. Hyg., 23:*27 (1974).

57. Nilsson, L. A., Betchlai, B., and Elwing, H. *Am. J. Trop. Med. Hyg., 29:*524 (1980).

58. Ambroise-Thomas, P., and Kien Truong, T. *Bull. W.H.O., 40:*103 (1969).

59. Ambroise-Thomas, P., and Kien Truong, T. *Am. J. Trop. Med. Hyg., 21:*907 (1972).

60. Thomas, V., Sinniah, B., and Leng, Y. P. *Am. J. Trop. Med. Hyg., 30:*57 (1981).

61. Bos, H. J., Van den Eijk, A. A., and Steerenberg, P. A. *Trans. Roy. Soc. Trop. Med. Hyg., 69:*440 (1976).

62. Hartmann, D. P., Ghadirian, E., and Meerovitch, E. *J. Parasitol., 66:*344 (1980).

63. Yang, J., and Kennedy, M. T. *J. Clin. Microbiol., 10:*778 (1979).

64. Voller, A., Bartlett, A., and Bidwell, D. E. *Trans. Roy. Soc. Trop. Med. Hyg., 70:*98 (1976).

65. Lin, T. M., Halbert, S. P., Chiu, C. T., and Zarco, R. *J. Clin. Microbiol., 13:*646 (1981).

66. Bos, H. J., Schouten, W. J., Noordpool, H., Makbin, M., and Oostburg, B. F. J. *Am. J. Trop. Med. Hyg., 29:*358 (1980).

67. Tandon, A. *Trans. Roy. Soc. Trop. Med. Hyg., 75:*574 (1981).

68. Williams, J. E., and Robinson, D. M. *Trans. Roy. Soc. Trop. Med. Hyg., 76:*280 (1982).

69. Root, D. M., Cole, F. X., Williamson, J. A. *Arch. Invest. Med., 9*(Suppl. 1):203 (1978).

70. Palacios, B., O., de la Hoz, R., and Sosa, H. *Arch. Invest. Med. (Mex)., 9*(Suppl. 1): 339 (1978).

71. Voller, A., Bidwell, D. E., Bartlett, A., and Edwards, R. *Trans. Roy. Soc. Trop. Med. Hyg., 71:*431 (1977).

72. Center for Disease Control. *Morb. Mort. Weekly Rep., 27:*167 (1978).

73. Rendtorff, R. C. *Am. J. Hyg., 59:*209 (1954).

74. Hartong, W. A., Gourley, W. K., and Arvanitakis, C. *Gastroenterology, 77:*61 (1979).

75. Filice, F. P. *Univ. of Calif. Publications in Zool., 57:*53 (1952).

76. Meyer, E. A., and Jarroll, E. L. *Am. J. Epidem., 111:*1 (1980).

77. Ackers, J. P. *Trans. Roy. Soc. Trop. Med. Hyg., 74:*427 (1980).

78. Meyer, E. A. *Experiment. Parasit., 39:*101 (1976).

79. Visvesvera, G. S. *Trans. Roy. Soc. Trop. Med. Hyg., 74:*213 (1980).

80. Gillin, F. D., and Diamond, L. S. *J. Parasitol., 66:*350 (1980).

81. Warhurst, D. C., and Wright, S. G. *Trans. Roy. Soc. Trop. Med. Hyg., 73:*601 (1979).

82. Moody, A. H. *Trans. Roy. Soc. Trop. Med. Hyg., 70:*338 (1976).

83. Danciger, M., and Lopez, M. *Am. J. Trop. Med. Hyg., 24:*237 (1975).

84. Beal, C. B., Viens, P., Grant, R. G. L., and Hughes, J. M. *Am. J. Trop. Med. Hyg., 19:*349 (1970).

85. Thomas, G. E., Goldsmid, J. M., and Wicks, A. C. B. *S. Afr. Med. J., 48:*2219 (1974).

86. Smith, P. D., Gillin, F. D., Brown, W. R., and Nash, T. E. *Gastroenterology, 80:*1476 (1981).

87. Wolfe, M. S. *N. Eng. J. Med., 298:*319 (1978).

88. Kamath, K. R., and Murugasu, R. *Gastroenterology, 66:*16 (1974).

89. Halita, M., and Isaicu, L. *Andealul Medical, 6:*154 (1946).

90. Ridley, M. J., and Ridley, D. S. *J. Clin. Path., 29:*30 (1976).

91. Wright, S. G., Moody, H. H., Tomkins, A. M., and Ridley, D. S. *Gut. 18:*986 (1977).

92. Visvesvara, G. S., Smith, P. D., Healy, G. R., and Brown, W. R. *Ann. Int. Med., 93:*802 (1980).

93. Ganguly, N. K., Mahajan, R. C., Vasudev, V., Krishna, V. R., Anand, B. S., Dilawari, J. B., and Chandanani, R. E. *Ind. J. Med. Res., 73*(Suppl): 111 (1981).

94. Roberts-Thomson, I. C., Steven, D. P., Mahmoud, A. A. F., and Warren, K. S. *Gastroenterology, 71:*57 (1976).

95. Vinayak, V. K., Jain, P., and Naik, S. R. *Ann. Trop. Med. Parasit., 72:*581 (1978).

96. Purpon, I., Jimenez, D., and Engelking, R. L. *J. Urol., 98:* 372 (1967).

97. Kacker, P. P. *Brit. J. Vener. Dis., 49:*318 (1973).

98. Shookhoff, H. B. *J. Am. Med. Ass., 222:*1310 (1972).

99. Lynch, B. deP. *J. Am. Med. Ass., 222:*1309 (1972).

100. Abrahm, P. M. *J. Am. Med. Ass., 222:*917 (1972).

101. Kean, B. H. *N. Y. State J. Med., 76:*930 (1976).

102. Dritz, A. K., Ainsworth, T. E., Garrard, W. F., Beck, A., Palmer, R. D., Boucher, L. A., and River, E. *Lancet 2:*3 (1977).

103. Meyers, J. D., Kuharic, H. A., and Holmes, K. K. *Brit. J. Vener. Dis., 53:*54 (1977).

104. William, D. C. *Cutis, 27:*278 (1981).

105. Personal communication, Ms. Bernadine Flejzor, Roosevelt Hospital, New York City.

106. Personal communication, Pearl Ma, Ph.D., St. Vincent's Hospital, and Rose Maria Soave, M.D., New York University, New York City.

107. Hurwitz, A. L., and Owen, R. L. *West J. Med., 128:*89 (1978).

108. Mildvan, D., Gelb, A. M., and William, D. *J. Am. Med. Ass., 238:*1387 (1977).

109. Kazal, H. L., Sohn, N., Carrasco, J. I., Robilotti, J. G., Jr., and Delaney, W. E. *Ann. Clin. Lab. Sci., 6:*184 (1976).

110. Keystone, J. S., Keystone, D. L., and Proctor, E. M. *Can. Med. Ass. J., 123:*512 (1980).

111. Personal observation, J. D. Frame, M.D.

112. Levine, N. D. *Protozoan Parasites of Domestic Animals and Man,* 2nd Ed., Burgess, Minneapolis, 1973, p. 380, 385.

113. Reese, N. C., Current, W. L., Ernst, J. V., and Bailey, W. S. *Am. J. Trop. Med. Hyg., 31:*226 (1982).

114. Centers for Disease Control. *Morb. and Mort. Wkly. Repts., 31:*252 (1982).

115. Centers for Disease Control. *Morb. and Mort. Wkly. Repts., 30:*305 (1981).

8

Viral Gastroenteritis

NEIL R. BLACKLOW and GEORGE CUKOR
Division of Infectious Diseases
University of Massachusetts Medical School
Worcester, Massachusetts

Recently, rapid progress has occurred in our understanding of the etiology of viral gastroenteritis. Unlike the situation with most other viral infections, the major etiologic agents of this common syndrome are not diagnosed by their replication in cell cultures or laboratory animals. Rather, the viral gastroenteritis agents of major medical importance are diagnosed through their detection directly in stool specimens, using electron microscopic or immunologic techniques. The most striking recent advances in the diagnosis of viral gastroenteritis have occurred with the development of highly sensitive, specific, and rapid solid-phase immunoassay techniques. This chapter will concentrate on a review and analysis of these assays because they are the diagnositc techniques of choice for most laboratories. However, in order to facilitate a discussion of the immunoassays for the diagnosis of viral gastroenteritis agents, clinical, epidemiologic, and virologic background information relevant to this syndrome will first be reviewed.

I. BACKGROUND INFORMATION ON VIRAL GASTROENTERITIS

Acute viral gastroenteritis is an extremely common illness that affects all age groups and occurs in both epidemic and endemic forms (6). It is second in frequency only to the common cold among illnesses affecting United States families under epidemiological surveillance. It is also responsible for some of the common travelers' diarrhea encountered in Latin America, Africa, and Asia. The illness varies in its clinical presentation, but in general it is self-limited, begins with an explosive onset, and consists of varying combinations of diarrhea, nausea, vomiting, low grade fever, abdominal cramps, headache, anorexia, myalgia and malaise. It can be severe, indeed fatal, in the elderly, infant, debilitated or malnourished patient.

Viral gastroenteritis occurs primarily in two epidemiologically distinct clinical forms (6). One entity is usually sporadic and occasionally epidemic and it occurs predominantly in infants and young children (6). This form of illness typically produces severe diarrhea that commonly lasts for five to eight days and is usually accompanied by fever and vomiting. Rotavirus, which was discovered during the 1970's (2), is responsible for approximately one half of the cases of this clinical entity world-wide requiring hospitalization. Although the major target of rotavirus is the very young, it can produce clinical disease in adults but the infection is most commonly subclinical in this age group. Rotavirus is 70nm in diameter, possesses a double shelled outer capsid, and is a member of the Reoviridae family of viruses. The virus was originally discovered and has been easily identified by routine electron microscopy in stool filtrates derived from ill individuals (15). Serologic assay techniques have been developed for this agent and can detect antibodies in human sera (3). In addition, rotavirus has been identified in diarrheal feces by immunologic assays such as RIA or enzyme-linked immunosorbent assay (EIA) techniques (8,13,38). Available laboratory techniques have readily permitted in vitro study of the biologic properties of rotavirus and have shown that it possesses double stranded segmented RNA. The etiologic role of rotavirus in diarrheal illness has been demonstrated in many parts of the world, and in addition to pediatric and family settings has also been associated with diarrhea experienced by adults including travelers (9,30,32). Recently, some but not all strains of human rotavirus have been cultivated in cell culture by incorporating low concentrations of trypsin into the culture medium (25,27) and blind passaging the inoculated cell cultures several times. At least three and perhaps as many as five serotypes of human rotavirus exist (28,34). Interestingly, human rotaviruses are closely related immunologically to other animal rotaviruses, some of which grow readily in cell culture unlike the human virus, and this feature has been exploited for clinical diagnostic purposes (8,23). Rotavirus is detectable in feces during acute illness and is usually shed for up to 8 days after onset of symptoms and occasionally longer. Nosocomial spread of infection among hospitalized pediatric patients and medical personnel is well documented.

The second clinical entity is characteristically epidemic and is responsible for family and community-wide outbreaks of gastroenteritis among older children and adults (6). The older medical literature gives a variety of descriptive labels to this one to two day illness, such as winter vomiting disease, epidemic collapse, viral diarrhea, epidemic diarrhea and vomiting, and acute infectious nonbacterial gastroenteritis. Recently, a newly discovered agent, Norwalk virus, has been shown to be responsible for about 40 percent of these disease outbreaks in the United States (17).

Other Norwalk-like viruses have also been discovered such as Hawaii agent and W agent, and although they have not yet been studied epidemiologically, they are likely to be responsible for many more epidemic cases of this illness (6). The Norwalk-like viruses are of uncertain classification and were originally discovered through human volunteer studies in which gastroenteritis was transmitted by the oral administration of bacteria-free, toxin-free stool filtrates derived from several outbreaks of the disease (6). The prototype Norwalk virus, which is still currently noncytopathic in vitro and not disease producing for experimental animals, was subsequently visualized in infectious stool filtrates and partially characterized as a 27nm small particle of definable density by immune electron microscopy (IEM) and ultracentrifugation (14). Other Norwalk-like viruses, such as Hawaii and Ditchling viruses, have been uncovered by similar techniques; these two agents appear to form (with Norwalk virus) three immunologically distinct agents based on IEM studies (6,33). Both the Norwalk and Hawaii agents produce a mucosal lesion of the proximal human small intestine, the likely site for replication of these viruses (26). This lesion is accompanied by transient small intestinal malabsorption, and also by delayed gastric emptying despite normal gastric morphology and secretory function (20). A radioimmunoassay (RIA) technique has been developed for the detection of Norwalk virus in diarrheal stools and for quantitation of antibody to the agent (4,11). It relies upon clinical materials derived from human volunteer studies since it has not been possible to prepare hyperimmune animal serum to the virus. The RIA procedure has been used to demonstrate the epidemiologic importance of Norwalk virus in various parts of the world, including its involvement in waterborne, foodborne, nursing home, and school and community outbreaks of acute gastroenteritis (17). The virus has also been associated with cases of travelers' diarrhea (9,18). RIA procedures do not exist for the other Norwalk-like viruses.

During the past few years, several other agents of viral gastroenteritis have been described, including enteric adenovirus, calicivirus, enteric coronavirus, and astrovirus (6). The medical importance of these agents is currently not known, in contrast to Norwalk virus and rotavirus.

II. RATIONALE FOR USE OF SOLID PHASE IMMUNOASSAYS FOR DIAGNOSIS OF ROTAVIRUS

The detection of rotavirus in a diarrheal stool specimen is the procedure necessary for making the diagnosis in an individual patient (5,15). Although serologic assays demonstrating antibody seroconversions are helpful in epidemiologic studies, they do not provide information for rapid diagnosis during illness; in addition, detectable pre-existing rotavirus antibodies are found in most individuals because of the ubiquitous nature of the virus (6,15). A rapid diagnosis of rotavirus illness helps to provide the clinician with a reliable prognosis for the patient, may prevent unnecessary use of antimicrobial therapy and prolonged hospitalization, and permits institution of appropriate control measures.

Despite the recent success in cultivation of human rotavirus in cell culture, this procedure is time-consuming, cumbersome, and currently only allows for the growth of approximately 50% of isolates. Thus, in vitro cultivation of the virus should be considered as an exciting research tool but not a practical diagnostic technique. As for electron microscopy, this procedure resulted in the original discovery of rotavirus and it was initially used extensively for rotavirus diagnosis. It still is used in some laboratories today. It remains the standard by which other assays must be evaluated (15). However, the usefulness of EM is limited in practical terms by the requirement for highly specialized equipment and personnel as well as by the difficulty in handling large numbers of specimens.

Thus, EM has been replaced in most laboratories by solid phase immunoassays which are the diagnostic tests of choice for most situations (5,15). The immunoassay offers same day or next day diagnosis of rotavirus infection and can be performed on a large scale with routinely available equipment and personnel. In this assay, the stool specimen to be tested is exposed to a solid phase which has first been coated with antirotavirus antibody. After an absorption period and washing, a labeled virus specific detection antibody is employed to demonstrate the presence of rotavirus bound to the solid phase.

Certain immunological characteristics of human rotavirus are pertinent to an understanding of the diagnostic immunoassay. Based on virus neutralization assays, at least 3 serotypes of rotavirus have been identified (28,34). Also, two additional different antigenic specificities, designated as subgroups, have been recognized by differential reactivity of virus strains in immunoassays (16). However, all human rotaviruses appear to have the same clinical and epidemiological patterns; therefore, grouping or typing of isolates currently serves no practical diagnostic use except to follow epidemiologic trends of infection. All mammalian rotaviruses, however, possess a common group specific antigen and several of the animal rotaviruses grow easily to high titer in cell culture. This fact can be exploited for the immunoassay by the use of these animal rotaviruses as purified antigens for the preparation of hyperimmune diagnostic sera (8).

III. CRITICAL FACTORS IN PERFORMANCE OF ROTAVIRUS IMMUNOASSAYS

There are several factors that must be taken into consideration for the performance of solid phase immunoassays for the detection of rotavirus in stools. These include the selection of serum reagents, solid phase, stool sample preparation, test conditions, indicator system, direct vs. indirect assay, specificity controls and method of calculating results. These factors shall now be reviewed because they are critically important for the proper performance and interpretation of the rotavirus immunoassay.

A. Reagent Sera For Use as Coating and Detection Antibodies

Selection of these reagent sera represents perhaps the most critical step in the establishment of the immunoassay. Convalescent human sera are not of sufficiently high titer for practical use and therefore hyperimmune animal sera need to be used. Three general approaches have been employed for the preparation of diagnostic hyperimmune antirotavirus serum. The first approach involves the purification of human rotavirus directly from human feces and then its use as antigen for the immunization of laboratory animals (10, 19,21,22,24). The serious problem with this approach is that the hyperimmune serum produced may contain antibody reactive with human stool components which copurified with the virus. The end result is high background reactions and even false positive results with some stools which happen to contain high concentrations of the reacting antigen. The second approach takes advantage of the ability of human rotavirus to induce illness in gnotobiotic newborn calves. Rotavirus is then purified from calf feces, thereby avoiding contamination with human antigenic stool components and permitting its use as an immunogen (13,35). The third approach is the most practical one and takes advantage of the rotavirus group specific antigen by using a cell culture derived animal rotavirus as the immunogen for preparation of hyperimmune serum (8,12,23). Simian rotavirus, SA-11, and calf rotavirus, NCDV, have been most commonly used for this purpose. Because of its relative simplicity and avoidance of fecally derived virus as an immunogen, the third approach is currently preferred by most laboratories.

In addition, it is preferable that the coating and detection antibodies be prepared in different animal species in order to obviate additional problems associated with non-specific reactivity of serum reagents. This is because any undesired reactivity present in only one of the reagent serums will not interfere with the immunoassay. Animals successfully used for preparation of hyperimmune rotavirus serum have been guinea pigs, goats, and rabbits. It should also be noted that not all individual animals within a single species produce satisfactory serum, and thus several animals should be immunized and their sera tested separately in the immunoassay (8).

B. Solid Phase

Microtiter plates made of flexible polyvinyl chloride have been used with goat serum as the coating antibody. With other animal sera, hard polystyrene plates may also be used. Individual polystyrene beads coated with antibody can be employed advantageously if small or variable numbers of specimens are to be tested.

C. Processing of Stool Specimens for Testing

Acute illness diarrheal stools are the only specimens likely to contain rotavirus-specific antigen; these specimens can be stored unaltered at -70°C if desired by the laboratory. When stools are to be tested, no serum should be used in the diluent for the stools unless it is first shown to be negative for rotavirus antibody. One method for processing stools involves preparation of a 2 to 10% stool suspension in veal infusion broth supplemented with 0.5% bovine serum albumin, followed by mixing and clarification with low speed centrifugation (5). Rectal swab specimens are adequate for testing but less satisfactory than stool specimens.

D. General Test Conditions

Numerous test conditions are reported, and it appears that the incubation conditions are not critical if high titered reagents are used at optimal concentrations predetermined by checkerboard titration (1,40). Incubation periods have usually lasted 1 to 12 hours at 37°C or room temperature.

E. Selection of RIA or EIA Indicator System

Labeling of the detection antibody for the immunoassay can be either with radioiodine or an enzyme, resulting in RIA or EIA tests, respectively. RIA is satisfactory only in a very large diagnostic laboratory or a research laboratory where numerous specimens are to be tested and iodination facilities are available. This is because of the need for handling and disposing of radioactive materials. Furthermore the radiolabeled antibody has a relatively short shelf life. In contrast, EIA is more practical for most diagnostic laboratories (41). In EIA, the detection antibody is conjugated to an enzyme such as alkaline phosphatase, horseradish peroxidase, or beta-galactosidase. When a chromogenic substrate is added, bound antibody may be quantitated using a spectrophotometer. Spectrophotometers are now available that have been modified for use in EIA tests.

F. Configuration of the Assay: Direct versus Indirect

The direct test immunoassay consists of first a coating antibody attached to the solid phase, followed by the stool specimen to be tested, and followed lastly by the labeled virus-specific detection antibody. The indirect test inserts an extra step after the test stool specimen is added (36). An unlabeled antirotavirus serum, derived from an animal species other than the source of the coating antibody, is added after the stool specimen. Lastly, a labeled antiglobulin directed against the animal species of the second antibody is employed as the detection antibody. The indirect assay has the advantage of a laboratory being able to use a single labeled antiglobulin for many different types of immunoassays, rather than having to label each detection antibody. When properly controlled, the indirect assay has been used successfully for the detection of rotavirus, with results comparable to the direct assay (7,24,38).

Although indirect tests have a theoretical advantage of increased sensitivity, this has not proven to be the case with rotavirus immunoassays (12). This is probably due to the high titers of rotavirus shed in diarrheal stools from pediatric patients (29), which suffice to render the direct assay sensitive for diagnostic purposes. Thus, since it has one less step to be performed, the direct assay for rotavirus is more convenient than the indirect assay. Moreover, reports have indicated that the indirect test has an increased incidence of nonspecific reactions as well as high background levels of reaction, resulting in reduced sensitivity and specificity (7,12,24,36). These problems are discussed in the following section.

G. Specificity of the Assay and Use of Controls

Serious problems occurred with the specificity of the original immunoassays for rotavirus, which have subsequently been overcome. Originally, the positivity of test stool specimens was determined by their comparison with reactions obtained with a panel of known negative stool samples (13,35). Borderline positive specimens were subjected to a confirmatory test, consisting of exogenous blocking (neutralization) of sample reactivity by a high titered antirotavirus serum. In practice in research laboratories, the confirmatory test was infrequently used. In time, however, it became apparent that there were serious difficulties with the frequency of non-specific reactions (7,36,37). Initially, it was noted that stools from individuals living in certain geographic areas possessed nonspecific activity against goat serum, which was speculated to relate to their diet. It was also noted that other stools contained non-specific antiglobulin activity related to an IgM molecule in the stools. Accordingly, normal goat serum and a reducing agent were added to all fecal samples to cope with these problems (37). In addition, EDTA or bovine serum albumin have been added to stools and test samples have had their pH neutralized in order to try to eliminate nonspecific reactions (12,21). These procedures reduced but did not totally eliminate all nonspecific reactions. In an extensive study from Washington, D.C. (7), it was found that nearly three-quarters of 1,834 tests originally felt to be positive by indirect EIA could not be confirmed by EM, blocking EIA, confirmatory EIA or a combination of these methods. This high rate of false-positive EIA reactions was postulated to be in part due to nonspecific binding of rotavirus antibody to intestinal bacteria or their products such as staphylococcal protein A.

As a result of these problems a new test system has been devised which avoids the inadequacies of measures such as adding reducing agent to stools, using known negative stools as controls, or testing borderline stool specimens by blocking reaction. In this new test system, originally used for Norwalk virus detection (11), a confirmatory test is automatically included for each sample (15,38). Thus, the reaction of a test stool specimen with rotavirus-positive serum is compared with the reaction of the same stool specimen with control rotavirus-negative (pre-immunization) serum. When this new test system was used by the Washington, D.C. group in an indirect EIA, false-positive results failed to occur (7).

H. Method of Calculating Results

Several methods exist to calculate the borderline between positive and negative samples. In RIA tests, positive/negative (P/N) values are usually calculated by dividing the radioactivity bound to the rotavirus positive serum containing microwell by the radioactivity bound to the rotavirus negative serum containing microwell. P/N values greater than 2 are then usually considered to be positive (8,13). In EIA tests, a P minus N calculation is often used because control absorbance values may be lower and more variable (23,35). The method of calculation of results should be validated for each new assay developed, by testing large numbers of known positive and negative specimens and comparing results with an established standard, usually EM (1,7,8,10,12,13,19,21-24,31,35,39).

I. Prepared EIA Tests Available for Rotavirus

As of this writing, one EIA test for rotavirus is commercially available and additional ones are anticipated. Abbott's "Rotazyme" assay is a direct test that uses polysytrene beads, and guinea pig and rabbit anti-SA11 rotavirus sera (23). The test apparently has special formulations of sample diluent and wash solutions that are sufficient to overcome most false positive results; the assay lacks a confirmatory test. The "Rotazyme" seems to possess favorable sensitivity and specificity for the testing of pediatric stool samples. A laboratory using the test may choose also to employ an exogenous confirmatory blocking test with any high titered antirotavirus serum in conjunction with the "Rotazyme."

IV. RADIOIMMUNOASSAY FOR DIAGNOSIS OF NORWALK VIRUS

Diagnostic procedures for Norwalk virus have lagged far behind those for rotavirus. There are several reasons for this. Norwalk virus is quite small (27nm) and can only be visualized by the laborious and technically difficult procedure of immuneelectron microscopy (IEM) (14). Furthermore, the virus is shed in relatively small amounts in stools, and has yet to be cultivated in vitro or in laboratory animals (6). Unlike rotavirus, no immunologically related substitute antigen is available. Also, highly purified virus has not been prepared from feces and thus hyperimmune animal sera useful for diagnostic purposes are not available.

Currently, an RIA procedure is available for the detection of Norwalk virus in stools and for the quantitation of antibodies to the virus in sera and intestinal fluids (4,11). Unfortunately, the RIA test is limited to just a few research laboratories that possess the necessary diagnostic reagents. These reagents are serum and stool samples derived from human volunteers who have been infected with Norwalk virus. Volunteers are currently the only model system for the study of the pathogenesis of Norwalk virus infection. Clearly, an assay for Norwalk virus that would be widely available and would avoid the use of human derived reagents is greatly needed, particularly by diagnostic laboratories and public health authorities seeking the cause of gastroenteritis epidemics.

The principle of the RIA test for the detection of Norwalk virus is similar to that of the confirmatory RIA test for rotavirus described above. Separate wells of microtiter plates are coated with acute and convelscent phase sera from a volunteer who has previously developed Norwalk virus illness. After addition of the test stool specimen, convalescent phase serum from a second volunteer is employed as a radioiodine labeled detection antibody. This procedure may be modified into a blocking test for the quantitation of antibody by the addition of the test specimen into the procedure outlined above after a known positive stool sample has been added.

REFERENCES

1. Beards, G. M., Bryden, A. S.: Evaluation of a new enzyme-linked immunosorbent assay test for rotavirus antigen in faeces. *J. Clin. Pathol. 34:*1388-1391, 1981.

2. Bishop, R. F., Davidson, G. P., Holmes, I. H., Ruck, B. J.: Virus particles in epithelial cells of duodenal mucosa from children with acute nonbacterial gastroenteritis. *Lancet ii:* 1281-1283, 1973.

3. Blacklow, N. R., Echeverria, P., Smith, D. H.: Serologic studies with reovirus-like enteritis agent. *Infection & Immunity 13:* 1563-1566, 1976.

4. Blacklow, N. R., Cukor, G., Bedigian, M. K., Echeverria, P., Greenberg, H. B., Schreiber, D. S., Trier, J. S.: Immune response and prevalence of antibody to Norwalk enteritis virus as determined by radioimmunoassay. *J. Clin. Microbiol. 10:*903-909, 1979.

5. Blacklow, N. R., Cukor, G.: Viral gastroenteritis agents. *Manual of Clinical Microbiology* 3rd ed., eds. E. H. Lennette, A. Balows, W. Hausler, J. Truant (American Society for Microbiology, Washington, D.C.), pp. 891-898, 1980.

6. Blacklow, N. R., Cukor, G.: Viral gastroenteritis. *New England J. Medicine 304:*397-406, 1981.

7. Brandt, C. D., Kim, H. W., Rodriguez, W. J., Thomas, L., Yolken, R. H., Arrobio, J. O., Kapikian, A. Z., Parrott, R. H., Chanock, R. M. Comparison of direct electron microscopy, immune electron microscopy, and rotavirus enzyme-linked immunosorbent assay for detection of gastroenteritis viruses in children. *J. Clinical Microbiology 13:*976-981, 1981.

8. Cukor, G., Berry, M. K., Blacklow, N. R. Simplified radioimmunoassay for detection of human rotavirus in stools. *J. Inf. Dis., 138:*906-910, 1978.

9. Echeverria, P., Blacklow, N. R., Sanford, L. B., Cukor, G.: Travelers' diarrhea among American Peace Corps volunteers in rural Thailand. *J. Inf. Dis., 143:*767-771, 1981.

10. Grauballe, P. C., Vestergaard, B. F., Meyling, A., Genner, J.: Optimized enzyme-linked immunosorbent assay for detection of human and bovine rotavirus in stools. Comparison with electron-microscopy, immunoelectro-osmophoresis, and fluorescent antibody techniques. *J. Medical Virology 7:*29-40, 1981.

11. Greenberg, H. B., Wyatt, R. G., Valdesuso, J., Kalica, A. R., London, W. T., Chanock, R. M., Kapikian, A. Z.: Solid-phase microtiter radioimmunoassay for detection of the Norwalk strain of acute nonbacterial epidemic gastroenteritis virus and its antibodies. *J. Med. Virol. 2:*97-108, 1978.

12. Hammond, G. W., Ahluwalia, G. S., Barker, F. G., Horsman, G., Hazelton, P. R.: Comparison of direct and indirect enzyme immunoassays with direct ultracentrifugation before electron microscopy for detection of rotaviruses. *J. Clinical Microbiology 16:*53-59, 1982.

13. Kalica, A. R., Purcell, R. H., Sereno, M. M., Wyatt, R. G., Kim, H. W., Chanock, R. M., Kapikian, A. Z.: A microtiter solid phase radioimmunoassay for detection of the human reovirus-like agent in stools. *J. Immunology 118:*1275-1279, 1977.

14. Kapikian, A. Z., Wyatt, R. G., Dolin, R., Thornhill, T. S., Kalica, A. R., Chanock, R. M.: Visualization by immune electron microscopy of a 27nm particle associated with acute infectious nonbacterial gastroenteritis. *J. Virol., 10:*1075-1081, 1972.

15. Kapikian, A. Z., Yolken, R. H., Greenberg, H. B., Wyatt, R. G., Kalica, A. R., Chanock, R. M., Kim, H. W.: Gastroenteritis viruses. In E. H. Lennette and N. J. Schmidt (ed.) Diagnostic procedures for viral, rickettsial and chlamydial infections. American Public Health Association, Washington, D.C., 1979, pp. 927-955.

16. Kapikian, A. Z., Cline, W. L., Greenberg, H. B., Wyatt, R. G., Kalica, A. R., Banks, C. E., James, H. D., Flores, J., Chanock, R. M.: Antigenic characterization of human and animal rotaviruses by immune adherence hemagglutination assay (IAHA): evidence for distinctness of IAHA and neutralization antigens. *Infection and Immunity 33:*415-425, 1981.

17. Kaplan, J. E., Gary, G. W., Baron, R. C., Singh, N., Schonberger, L. B., Feldman, R., Greenberg, H. B.: Epidemiology of Norwalk gastroenteritis and the role of Norwalk virus in outbreaks of acute nonbacterial gastroenteritis. *Ann. Int. Med., 96:*756-761, 1982.

18. Kesswick, B. H., Blacklow, N. R., Cukor, G., DuPont, H. L., Vollet, J. J. Norwalk virus and rotavirus in travellers' diarrhea in Mexico. *The Lancet 1:*109-110, 1982.

19. Kjeldsberg, E., Mortensson-Egnund, K.: Comparison of solid-phase immune electron microscopy, direct-electron microscopy and enzyme-linked immunosorbent assay for detection of rotavirus in faecal samples. *J. Virological Methods 4:*45-53, 1982.

20. Meeroff, J. C., Schreiber, D. S., Trier, J. S., Blacklow, N. R.: Abnormal gastric motor function in viral gastroenteritis. *Ann. Int. Med., 22:*370-373, 1980.

21. Middleton, P. J., Holdaway, M. D., Petric, M., Szymanski, M. T., Tam, J. S.: Solid phase radioimmunoassay for the detection of rotavirus. *Infection and Immunity 16:*439-444, 1977.

22. Obert, G., Gloeckler, R., Burckard, J., Regenmortel, M. H. V.: Comparison of immunosorbent electron microscopy, enzyme immunoassay and counterimmunoelectrophoresis for detection of human rotavirus in stools. *J. Virological Methods 3:*99-107, 1981.

23. Rubenstein, A. S., Miller, M. F.: Comparison of an enzyme immunoassay with electron microscopic procedures for detecting rotavirus. *J. Clin. Microbiol. 15:*938-944, 1982.

24. Sarkkinen, H. K., Halonen, P. E., Arstila, P. P.: Comparison of four-layer radioimmunoassay and electron microscopy for detection of human rotavirus. *J. Medical Virology 4:*255-260, 1979.

25. Sato, K., Inaba, Y., Shinozaki, T., Fujil, R., Matumoto, M.: Isolation of human rotavirus in cell cultures. *Archives Virology 69:*155-160, 1981.

26. Schreiber, D. S., Blacklow, N. R., Trier, J. S.: The mucosal lesion of the proximal small intestine in acute infectious nonbacterial gastroenteritis. *New Eng. J. Med., 288:*1318-1323, 1973.

27. Urasawa, T., Urasawa, S., Taniguchi, K.: Sequential passages of human rotavirus in MA-104 cells. *Microbiol. Immunol., 25:* 1025-1035, 1981.

28. Urasawa, S., Urasawa, T., Taniguchi, K.: Three human rotavirus serotypes demonstrated by plaque neutralization of isolated strains. *Infection & Immunity,* in press.

29. Vesikari, T., Sarkkinen, H. K., Maki, M.: Quantitative aspects of rotavirus excretion in childhood diarrhoea. *Acta. Paediatr. Scand., 70:*717-721, 1981.

30. vonBonsdorff, C. H., Hovi, T., Makela, P.: Rotavirus infections in adults in association with acute gastroenteritis. *J. Med. Virol., 2:*21-28, 1978.

31. Wall, R. A., Mellars, B. J., Luton, P., Boulding, S.: Comparison of ELISA, SPACE, and electron microscopy for the routine diagnosis of rotavirus infection. *J. Clin. Pathol., 35:*104-106, 1982.

32. Wenman, W. M., Hinde, D., Feltham, S., Gurwith, M.: Rotavirus infection in adults: results of a prospective family study. *New Eng. J. Med., 301:*303-306, 1979.

33. Wyatt, R. G., Greenberg, H. B., Kalica, A. R., Chanock, R. M., Kapikian, A.Z.: Structural and physicochemical properties of small enteric viruses. In Enteritis Virales/Viral Enteritis. Paris, France: Inserm. 1979; *90:*163-182.

34. Wyatt, R. G., Greenberg, H. B., James, W. D., Pittman, A. C., Kalica, A. R., Flores, J., Chanock, R. M., Kapikian, A.Z.: Definition of human rotavirus serotypes by plaque reduction assay. *Infection and Immunity 37:*110-115, 1982.

35. Yolken, R. H., Kim, H. W., Clem, T., Wyatt, R. G., Kalica, A. R., Chanock, R. M., Kapikian, A. Z.: Enzyme-linked immunosorbent assay (ELISA) for detection of human reovirus-like agent of infantile gastroenteritis. *Lancet ii:*263-267, 1977.

36. Yolken, R., Wyatt, R. G., Kapikian, A. Z.: Elisa for rotavirus. *Lancet ii:*819, 1977.

37. Yolken, R. H., Stopa, P. J.: Analysis of nonspecific reactions in enzyme-linked immunosorbent assay testing for human rotavirus. *J. Clin. Microbiol., 10:*703-707, 1979.

38. Yolken, R. H., Stopa, P. J., Harris, C. C.: Enzyme immunoassay for the detection of rotavirus antigen and antibody. In N. Rose and H. Friedman (ed). Manual of clinical immunology. 2nd ed. American Society for Microbiology, Washington, D.C., 692-699, 1980.

39. Yolken, R. H., Leister, F. J.: Evaluation of enzyme immunoassays for the detection of human rotavirus. *J. Inf. Dis., 144:*379, 1981.

40. Yolken, R. H., Leister, F. J.: Rapid multiple determinant enzyme immunoassay for the detection of human rotavirus. *J. Inf. Dis., 146:*43-46, 1982.

41. Yolken, R. H.: Enzyme immunoassays for the detection of infectious antigens in body fluids: current limitations and future prospects. *Reviews of Infectious Diseases, 4:*35-68, 1982.

9

Feces Culture: The Dilemma of the Clinical Microbiology Laboratory

ALEX C. SONNENWIRTH
Departments of Microbiology and Immunology, and Pathology
Washington University School of Medicine
Division of Microbiology
The Jewish Hospital of St. Louis
St. Louis, Missouri

In selecting topics for the 1978 Symposium on The Impact of Infections on Medical Care in the United States (4), Kunin listed as one of the major unsolved problems in clinical infectious disease "the procurement of reliable and relevant cultures .... and prompt, low cost reports on significant organisms (9)." The dilemma of the *relevant* and *reliable* feces culture is part of this overall problem.

A large number of "new" or "newer" bacterial entities involved in diarrheal diseases have been described recently, i.e., *Yersinia enterocolitica, Campylobacter fetus* ssp *jejuni, Vibrio parahaemolyticus* and other vibrios, enterotoxigenic *Escherichia coli*, and pseudomembranous enterocolitis involving *Clostridium difficile* or possibly *Staphylococcus aureus* (8). The question needs to be posed at this point: Where do we go from here in the clinical laboratory? How much do we do, and how far do we go with stool specimens?

The clinical microbiology laboratory is asked to deliver *rapid, reliable* and *relevant* results, in the *shortest* possible time, for the *lowest* possible price. It is thus necessary to center on discussing the feasibility of these goals, the possible approach of individual laboratories, and the obligation of microbiologists to educate physicians through truthful and relevant reporting of findings, or at least accurate reporting of what *was* or was *not* looked for.

Before proceeding, however, it should be useful to review briefly the general types of diarrheal illness resulting in submission of fecal specimens.

As shown in Table 1, the first type of diarrheal illness may be *drug-induced,* primarily involving clindamycin, but also other antimicrobials. The diarrhea may vary from mild to severe colitis with pseudomembrane formation. The role of *Clostridium difficile* has been recently elucidated (1). In addition, antimetabolites, and thyroid replacement can also cause diarrhea.

Common-source diarrhea (Table 2) usually involves a history of other persons with similar illness following common exposure (food, water).

When food-borne disease is suspected and none of those involved has a fever, a toxin-mediated illness should be suspected. With

Table 1.

DRUG-INDUCED DIARRHEA
CLINDAMYCIN, LINCOMYCIN OTHER ANTIMICROBIALS ANTIMETABOLITES THYROID REPLACEMENT
CLOSTRIDIUM DIFFICILE
STAPHYLOCOCCUS AUREUS

Table 2.

COMMON SOURCE DIARRHEA	
SALMONELLA	SHIGELLA
YERSINIA ENTEROCOLITICA VIBRIO (PARAHAEM., CHOLERAE)	CAMPYLOBACTER E. COLI
STAPHYLOCOCCUS; C. PERFRINGENS; (B. CEREUS)	
(PROTOZOA)	(VIRUSES)

very short incubation (2-4 hours), *staphylococcal food poisoning* is probable.

When onset is later than 12-16 hours after ingestion, *Clostridium perfringens* or other toxigenic bacteria may be involved.

If patient(s) has fever, likely causative agents may be *Salmonella, Shigella, Campylobacter, Yersinia enterocolitica,* or *Vibrio parahaemolyticus.*

It is highly important that the laboratory be apprised of patient's history and any suspicion the physician may entertain concerning patient's exposure.

Until very recently feces cultures were performed solely for the detection of *Salmonella* and *Shigella.* If not found, the laboratory usually reported: "No enteric pathogens found." This now is simply not adequate.

As discussed in the preceeding chapters, it is now possible to detect and identify *Y. enterocolitica, Campylobacter,* and vibrios in diarrheal stools. There are procedures for the determination of the toxigenicity of *E. coli* strains and for the detection of *C. difficile* toxins, and it is likely that immunological tests will soon appear that will allow performance of these determinations in the clinical laboratory.

Present ("routine") procedures. *Salmonella* and *Shigella* should be searched for in stool cultures (Table 3). This requires 2 or 3 media (differential and selective) as well as an enrichment broth.

The laboratory inspection and accreditation material of the College of American Pathologists continues to require routine use of differential media to allow recovery and identification of gram-positive cocci (staphylococci) and of yeasts in each and every stool culture. This requirement is debatable and is not followed by many laboratories.

The new Cumitech volume on laboratory diagnosis of diarrhea (6) does not require routine use of blood agar and Sabouraud plates for stool cultures.

Yersinia enterocolitica. (See Chapter 2.) For about a decade, *Yersinia enterocolitica* has been known to be a major enteric pathogen (2). Thousands of cases have been culturally proven in Europe and other continents; it is frequently isolated in Quebec from children with diarrhea, and has been involved in a major common-source outbreak in Oneida County in New York. However, its significance is still debated in the U.S., and it is described as being relatively rare.

Weissfeld and Sonnenwirth have recently reported (10) the incidence rate of *Y. enterocolitica* (2.1%) in an adult, hospitalized, symptomatic population in the U.S. Midwest as being equal to that of *Salmonella*, and more common than *Shigella*.

Procedures for detecting *Y. enterocolitica* in stools are shown in Table 4. The commonest approach has been to use duplicate MacConkey

Table 3.

"Routine" (Salmonella, Shigella)
MacConkey or EMB
HE, XLD, SS or DC
BS or BG
GN, selenite or tetrathio. broth

Table 4.

PARTIAL SCREEN:	
MacConkey duplicate plate	25° C
SS duplicate plate	25° C
CAL agar	25° C
COLD ENRICHMENT:	
Stool suspension (buff. saline)	4° C
Plate at 7, 14 and 21 days to: MacConkey, SS: 25° C	

and SS agar plates with incubation of one set at 35° C and another at room temperature. Cellobiose-arginine-lysine (CAL) as well as cefsulodin-irgasan-novobiocin agar (CIN) plates (7) have been highly successful in isolation of *Y. enterocolitica* from stools, as has cold enrichment; the latter, however, is too protracted for clinical usefulness. Other procedures, such as KOH treatment of stools (11) hold promise for easier isolation of *Y. enterocolitica*.

Stool culture for Y. enterocolitica. For routine procedure, inoculate plate of MacConkey (1 loopful) and 1 plate of SS agar (2 loopfuls) with stool; if possible, inoculate CAL plate also. Incubate plates at *25 C*, since *Y. enterocolitica* grows more readily on plates at 25 C than at 35 C.

In some laboratories the above 2 plates are inoculated as part of the routine stool culture; i.e., MacConkey and other enteric agars are inoculated and incubated at 35 C, with the 2 plates described above added to each stool culture, and incubated separately at room temperature, i.e., 22-25 C.

Cold enrichment. Y. enterocolitica proliferates at 4-5 C and presumably outgrows other enteric flora. The recovery of *Y. enterocolitica* is much more satisfactory using the cold enrichment technic than by direct plating of specimens. If possible, all sample material should be refrigerated from time of collection.

1. Place rectal swab or swab dipped in feces in test tube containing 5 ml of 0.067M phosphate buffered saline (PBS), pH 7.6, and hold tubes at 4-5C.

   The 0.067M PBS is prepared by mixing 8.5 g NaCl with 120 ml of 0.067M KH_2PO_4 and 880 ml of 0.067M Na_2HPO_4.

   a. Perform routine culture, as above (0 day culture).

   b. Hold cold enrichment specimens at 4-5 C for 3 wk. Place specimens on MacConkey and SS agar plates after 7, 14, and 21 d of enrichment. Incubate plates at 25 C.

Campylobacter. (See Chapter 1.) *C. fetus* ss *jejuni* has become known in the United States because of two 1978 gastroenteritis outbreaks in Vermont and Colorado (5). It is now isolated frequently in England, Canada, Belgium, and increasingly in the United States.

The organism is reasonably easy to grow in GasPak jar, Torbal jar, or with the Fortner principle (using a facultative organism to reduce oxygen in a plastic bag). With a new Oxoid supplement added to medium, it is claimed that it can be grown at 37° C instead of 42° (see Table 5).

Isolation of Campylobacter fetus ss. jejuni. Obtain feces or rectal swabs from individuals with diarrhea. If these can not be cultured within 4 hours, the rectal swabs or swabs containing feces are immersed in Cary Blair transport medium in screwtop vials.

1. Use rectal swabs or swab specimens of feces to inoculate area, approximately 1-1 1/4 in. in diameter, of surface of plate of selective medium (blood agar base no. 2--Oxoid, with 7% lysed horse blood and 3 antimicrobials, i.e., vancomycin, 10 μg/ml, polymyxin B, 2.5 I μ/ml, and trimethoprim, 5 μg/ml). Then streak plate to obtain isolated colonies.
2. Incubate plates at *42-43* C in anaerobic jar *with catalyst removed*; evacuate to 15 in. Hg twice, and refill each time with either of the following gas mixtures: (1) 10% carbon dioxide, 10% hydrogen, and 80% nitrogen; or (2) 5% carbon dioxide, 10% hydrogen, and 85% nitrogen. If facilities for gassing out an anaerobic jar are not available, a disposable GasPak hydrogen-carbon dioxide generator, *without catalyst,* may be substituted. Not all strains of *C. fetus* ssp. *jejuni* grow as well when GasPak generators are used, and some strains may not grow at all. *C. fetus* ssp. *jejuni* is a microaerophile, not a strict anaerobe; and

Table 5.

BRUCELLA BLOOD AGAR (BBA) - TRIMETHOPRIM, VANCOMYCIN, POLYMYXIN B: 42° C, GASPAK, TORBAL JAR, OR FORTNER PRINCIPLE
SAME, WITH SUPPLEMENT (OXOID SR85): CYCLOHEXIMIDE + BACITRACIN, COLISTIN, CEPHAZOLIN, NOVOBIOCIN, 37° C INCUBATION
THIOGLYCOLLATE WITH ANTIBIOTICS

3. Examine plates after 24, 48, and 72 h of incubation. Colonies of *C. fetus* ssp. *jejuni* are usually detectable by 24 hr. The colonies vary from pinpoint, glossy-appearing colonies to those that spread over entire surface of the agar.

Since *C. fetus* ssp. *jejuni* is an *oxidase-positive* organism, the *oxidase test* is used to screen suspect colonies.

Vibrios. (See Chapter 3.) *V. cholerae* is now isolated in the United States from nonimported cases, and *V. parahaemolyticus* also occurs in patients and contaminated foods (several outbreaks). Isolated cases of *V. parahaemolyticus* are rare, probably because the organism requires media with higher salt concentration (1.5%-3% (NaCl) than present in routine media. It is generally believed that this organism should be sought only in acute diarrheal illness *and* a history of seafood ingestion (however, there is some evidence in Japan and India that non-seafood may also contain *V. parahaemolyticus*).

Table 6 illustrates briefly the media required for isolation of *V. cholerae* and *V. parahaemolyticus*.

V. cholerae culture. Collect stool specimens within the first 24 hours of the disease. Rectal swabs can be used during the acute phase; during convalescence, swabs are not reliable. If

Table 6.

V. cholerae
Alkaline peptone water TCBS (or Monsur) agar
V. parahaemolyticus
Cary-Blair or alkaline peptone water TCBS agar XLD (or other selective medium) + 1.5% NaCl

specimens can not be cultured immediately or must be transported, inoculate alkaline peptone water (pH 8.4) and transport medium.

1. Stake out 1-2 loopfuls of stool on *TCBS* agar (inoculate heavily). Incubate 16-24 h at 35-37 C; and
2. Place 1-2 loopfuls of stool specimen into 0.5-1 ml *alkaline peptone water* (pH 8.4). Incubate 6-8 h at 37 C. Streak out plate as described above.

V. parahaemolyticus culture. Stools, rectal swabs, or vomitus specimens in outbreaks should be obtained at the earliest opportunity because the carrier state is short-lived.

1. If transit time is much beyond 8 hours:
   a. Place stool specimens in Cary-Blair transport medium.
   b. In laboratory, streak loopful onto TCBS agar in addition to other enteric media employed.
   c. Incubate at 35 C for 24-48 h.
   (Do not discard plates as negative before 48 h.)
2. If transit time is 8 hours or less:
   a. Place stool specimen in alkaline peptone water.
   b. After 8 h incubation, streak loopful onto TCBS agar.
   c. Incubate at 35 C for 24-48 h.
3. Rectal swab specimen:
   a. Sample specimen (preferably polyester fiber-tipped swab) contained in 7 ml medium (Cary-Blair or alkaline peptone water) by streaking loopful onto TCBS agar and other enteric agars.
   b. Incubate plates at 35 C for 24-48 h.

Clostridium difficile. (See Chapter 5.) In cases of suspected pseudomembranous enterocolitis (usually following antibiotic administration), it becomes necessary to determine presence of *C. difficile* toxin, a task presently only performed in a number of reference laboratories. Anaerobic culture for *C. difficile* can be best performed on the selective medium, CCFA (3), under anaerobic cultivation (Table 7). Other media containing antibiotics have also been used.

"Ideal" workup of feces. Table 8 summarizes the procedures to be done for an "ideal" workup of feces from a diarrheal patient: This would involve searching for *Salmonella, Shigella, Campylobacter, Y. enterocolitica,* and noncholera vibrios (if indicated).

Can all this be done? Obviously, each laboratory will have to decide for itself, based on: (a) variations of geographical incidence, if any, of these organisms, (b) patient population (pediatric vs. adult), (c) manpower, and (d) cost.

There is no doubt that input from the clinician is necessary for an optimal laboratory evaluation, such as age, travel history, and recent ingestion of certain foods. The laboratory can not blindly search for all possible pathogens in the stool.

Our dilemma then is the emergence of a number of "new" pathogens as against cost containment, cost effectiveness, and availability of hands. These two goals, namely the detection of etiologic agents as against the reduction of costs, are mutually

Table 7.

Cycloserine-cefoxitin-fructose-egg yolk agar (CCFA) 37° C - anaerobic
Lysed blood agar + kanamycin + menadione + haemin
Blood agar + nalidixic acid

Table 8.

I. SUSPECTED COMMON SOURCE DIARRHEA	
MacConkey	BBA + antibiotics,
HE, SS, or XLD	Thio + antibiotics
BS or BG	Alkaline peptone water
GN or others	TCBS, or XLD + 1.5% NaCl
MacConkey - 25°, SS - 25°; cold enrichment	
II. SUSPECTED DRUG-INDUCED DIARRHEA	
	Clostridium difficile - anaerobic culture (CCFA medium)
	Toxin Determination
	Mannitol salt agar
	Blood agar or PEA

exclusive and will strain decision making of the clinical laboratory to the utmost. Present diagnostic methods resulting in reports like "no enteric pathogens" or "no pathogens found" are no longer acceptable unless they include attempts for determining the presence of the newer pathogens. Present-day practice demands that every effort be made to routinely culture for *Campylobacter* and, using a simple screening procedure, for *Yersinia*. Whet there is a history of seafood ingestion, also culture for *Vibrio parahaemolyticus*.

Reports. If the laboratory's culture procedure consists only of screening for *Salmonella* and *Shigella*, and this is negative, the report should clearly state: "No *Salmonella* or *Shigella* isolated." Since many physicians are not aware of the special cultural requirements for the newer agents, it would be highly efficacious if the following would be added (as recommended by Dr. Raymond Bartlett, Hartford Hospital): "No *Salmonella* or *Shigella* isolated; please consult microbiology if symptoms persist or infection with

Yersinia, Staphylococcus aureus, Vibrio, Campylobacter, enterotoxigenic *E. coli* or *Clostridium difficile* is suspected." Thus, specific procedures would then be performed.

In laboratories where original culture of feces includes specific media and procedures for the newer agents (such as in the writer's laboratory), the report of a feces culture will reflect the exact findings and procedures, e.g. "No *Salmonella, Shigella, Campylobacter,* or *Yersinia* grown. Specimen not processed for *Vibrio* ssp. or *Clostridium difficile*." In this manner, the record accurately reflects the full extent of the work performed.

Summary. It is strongly recommended that wherever possible the scope of feces culture be extended beyond screening for *Salmonella* and *Shigella,* to encompass at least the detection of *Campylobacter fetus* ss. *jejuni* and of *Y. enterocolitica.* It is expected that more information will soon become available about the relative occurrence and incidence of these organisms in diarrheal disease.

REFERENCES

1. Bartlett, J. G. 1979. Antibiotic associated pseudomembranous colitis. Rev. Infect. Dis. 1:530-539.
2. Bottone, E. J. 1977. Yersinia enterocolitica: A panoramic view of a charismatic microorganism. CRC Crit. Rev. Microbiol. 5(2):211-241.
3. George, W. L., V. L. Sutter, D. Citron, and S. M. Finegold. 1979. Selective and differential medium for isolation of Clostridium difficile. J. Clin. Microbiol. 9:214-219.
4. Kunin, C. M., and R. Edelman. 1978. The impact of infections on medical care in the United States - Problems and priorities for future research. Ann. Intern. Med. 89:739-866.
5. Morbidity and Mortality Weekly Report 27(25):207-208; 226-227, 1978.
6. Sack, R. B., R. C. Tilton, and A. S. Weissfeld. 1980. Laboratory diagnosis of bacterial diarrhea (Rubin, S. G., Coord. Ed.). Cumulative Techniques and Procedures in Clinical Microbiology, No. 12. American Society for Microbiology, Washington, D.C.

7. Schiemann, D. A. 1979. Synthesis of a selective agar medium for Yersinia enterocolitica. Can. J. Microbiol. 25:1298-1304.

8. Sonnenwirth, A. C., and L. Jarett. 1980. Gradwohl's Clinical Laboratory Methods and Diagnosis, 8th ed. The C. V. Mosby Co., St. Louis, Missouri.

9. Sonnenwirth, A. C. 1978. Constraints under which the microbiology laboratory functions. Ann. Intern. Med. 89:785-788.

10. Weissfeld, A. S., and A. C. Sonnenwirth. 1980. Yersinia enterocolitica in adults with gastrointestinal disturbances: Need for cold enrichment. J. Clin. Microbiol. 11:196-197.

11. Weissfeld, A., and A. C. Sonnenwirth. 1981. Rapid isolation of Yersinia enteroc-litica from feces. Abstracts Annual Meeting, American Society for Microbiology.

Index